CRISIS WITHOUT END

CRISIS WITHOUT END

The Medical and Ecological Consequences of the Fukushima Nuclear Catastrophe

From the Symposium at the New York Academy of Medicine,
March 11–12, 2013

Edited By

Helen Caldicott

THE NEW PRESS

NEW YORK
LONDON

Requests for permission to reproduce selections from this book should be mailed to: Permissions Department, The New Press, 120 Wall Street, 31st floor, New York, NY 10005.

Published in the United States by The New Press, New York, 2014

Distributed by Perseus Distribution

LIBRARY OF CONGRESS CATALOGING-IN-PUBLICATION DATA

Crisis without end : the medical and ecological consequences of the Fukushima nuclear catastrophe / edited by Helen Caldicott.
    pages cm
"From the symposium at the New York Academy of Medicine, March 11-12, 2013."
Includes bibliographical references.
    ISBN 978-1-59558-960-6 (hardcover : alk. paper) -- ISBN 978-1-59558-970-5 (e-book) 1. Fukushima Nuclear Disaster, Japan, 2011. 2. Nuclear power plants--Accidents--Japan. I. Caldicott, Helen, editor.
  TK1365.J3C75 2014
  363.17'990952117--dc23
                                    2014023689

The New Press publishes books that promote and enrich public discussion and understanding of the issues vital to our democracy and to a more equitable world. These books are made possible by the enthusiasm of our readers; the support of a committed group of donors, large and small; the collaboration of our many partners in the independent media and the not-for-profit sector; booksellers, who often hand-sell New Press books; librarians; and above all by our authors.

www.thenewpress.com

Book design and composition by Bookbright Media
This book was set in Jansen Text

Printed in the United States of America

10 9 8 7 6 5 4 3 2 1

Contents

CRISIS WITHOUT END

Introduction

Helen Caldicott

O n March 11, 2011, an earthquake measuring nine on the
Richter scale struck off the east coast of Japan. Within
days, the ensuing tsunami had induced the meltdown of three
of the six nuclear reactors at the Fukushima Daiichi nuclear
power plant.

During the earthquake, the external power supply was lost
to the reactor complex. The pumps that circulate up to one
million gallons of water per minute to cool each reactor core
ceased to function. Emergency diesel generators situated below the plants kicked in, but these were soon swamped by the
tsunami. Without cooling, the radioactive cores in Units 1,
2, and 3 began to melt within hours. Over the next few days,
all three cores (each weighing up to one hundred tons) melted
their way through six inches of steel at the bottom of their
reactor vessels and oozed their way onto the concrete floor
of the containment buildings—a fact that the Japanese government and Tokyo Electric Power Company (TEPCO), the
power plant operator, continued to deny for months after the

disaster. At the same time the zirconium cladding covering thousands of uranium fuel rods reacted with water to create hydrogen, which initiated hydrogen explosions in Units 1, 2, 3, and 4.

Massive quantities of radiation escaped into the air and water: three times more noble gases (argon, xenon, and krypton) than at the Chornobyl nuclear power plant accident in 1986, and huge amounts of other volatile and nonvolatile radioactive elements, including cesium, tritium, iodine, strontium, silver, plutonium, americium, and rubidium.

Fukushima is now described as the greatest industrial accident in history.

The Japanese government considered plans to evacuate 35 million people from Tokyo as other reactors, including four at Fukushima Daini, several miles along the coast from Fukushima Daiichi, were also at risk. Meanwhile, thousands of people fled the area around the smoldering reactors, but they were not notified where the radioactive plumes were traveling despite the fact that there was a system in place to track the plumes. As a result, people fled directly into regions with the highest radiation concentrations, where they were exposed to high levels of whole-body external gamma radiation, inhaling radioactive air and swallowing radioactive elements.[1]

Administering inert potassium iodide to the exposed population would have blocked the uptake of radioactive iodine in their thyroid glands. Unfortunately, it was not supplied, except in the town of Miharu, where there was a conscientious mayor. Prophylactic iodine was, however, distributed to the staff of Fukushima Medical University in the days following the accident, after extremely high levels of radioactive iodine—1.9 million becquerels per kilogram—were discovered in leafy vegetables near the university.[2] Iodine contamination was already widespread in leafy vegetables and milk, while other isotopic contamination from substances such as cesium was widespread in vegetables, fruit, meat, milk, rice, and tea in many areas of Japan.[3]

The Fukushima disaster is not over and will not end for many millennia. The radioactive fallout, which has covered vast swaths of Japan, will remain toxic for hundreds of thousands of years. It cannot simply be "cleaned up," and it will continue to contaminate food, humans, and animals. It is unlikely that the three Fukushima Daiichi reactors that experienced total meltdowns will ever be disassembled or decommissioned. TEPCO claims such a massive undertaking will take them at least thirty to forty years. The International Atomic Energy Agency (IAEA) predicts that it will be more than forty years before any progress can be made because of the dangerous levels of radiation at these damaged reactors.

This accident is identical to the Chornobyl catastrophe in its medical implications. The Fukushima meltdowns will induce an epidemic of cancer as people ingest radioactive elements. The single meltdown and explosion at Chornobyl contaminated 40 percent of the European landmass. Already, according to a 2009 report published by the New York Academy of Sciences, over one million people have perished as a direct result of that catastrophe. Large parts of Europe will remain radioactive for hundreds of years, as will now be the case in Japan.[4]

In assessing the impact of the Fukushima disaster on Japan and on the planet, and in assessing the safety of nuclear power overall, it is imperative to understand and evaluate the biological and medical consequences of exposure to the kinds of radioactive elements that are released during an accident at a nuclear power plant.

THE MEDICAL IMPLICATIONS OF RADIATION

- **Fact One:** No dose of radiation is safe. Each dose received by the body is cumulative and adds to the risk of developing malignancy or genetic disease.
- **Fact Two:** Children are ten to twenty times more vulnerable to the carcinogenic effects of radiation than adults. Females tend to be more sensitive than males, while fetuses and immunocompromised patients are also extremely sensitive.
- **Fact Three:** High doses of radiation received from a nuclear meltdown (or from a nuclear weapon explosion) can cause acute radiation sickness, including hair loss, severe nausea, diarrhea, and bleeding. Reports of these illnesses—particularly among children—appeared within the first few months after the Fukushima accident.
- **Fact Four:** The latent period of carcinogenesis and the incubation time for leukemia is five to ten years.

For solid cancers, it is fifteen to eighty years. It has been shown that all modes of cancer can be induced by radiation exposure—both external and internal— as well as over six thousand genetic diseases caused by mutations in the eggs and sperm, which are passed on to future generations.

As we increase the level of background radiation in our environment—from medical procedures and X-ray scanning machines at airports to radioactive materials escaping from nuclear reactors and nuclear waste dumps—we will inevitably increase the incidence of cancer and genetic disease in future generations. A disaster such as what occurred at the Chornobyl and Fukushima nuclear power plants exponentially increases the risk of both cancer and genetic disease in exposed populations.

TYPES OF IONIZING RADIATION

There are five forms of ionizing radiation:

- **X-rays** are electromagnetic and cause mutations the instant they pass through a human body. X-rays are not emitted by radioactive materials, only from man-made medical equipment.
- **Gamma rays**, also electromagnetic, are emitted by many of the radioactive materials generated in nuclear reactors and by some naturally occurring radioactive elements in soil.

- **Alpha rays** are particulate and composed of two protons and two neutrons emitted from uranium atoms and other elements generated in reactors, such as plutonium, americium, curium, and einsteinium. Alpha particles travel a very short distance in the human body. They cannot penetrate the layers of dead skin in the epidermis to damage living skin cells. But when these radioactive elements enter the lungs, liver, bones, or other organs, they transfer a large dose of radiation over a long period of time to a very small volume of cells. Although most of these cells are killed, some on the edge of the radiation field remain alive. They are often mutated, potentially causing cancer. Alpha emitters are among the most carcinogenic materials known.
- **Beta rays**, like alpha rays, are also particulate. A beta ray is a charged electron emitted from a radioactive element, such as strontium-90, cesium-137, and iodine-131. The beta particle is light in mass, travels farther than an alpha particle, and also is mutagenic.
- **Neutron rays** are released during the fission process in a reactor or a bomb. Reactor 1 at Fukushima has been periodically emitting neutron radiation as sections of the molten core become intermittently critical. Neutrons are large radioactive particles that travel many kilometers. They pass through everything, including concrete and steel. There is no way to hide from them, and they are extremely mutagenic.

There are over two hundred radioactive elements, each with its own half-life, biological characteristics, and pathways in the food chain and the human body. Amazingly, most have never had their biological pathways examined. They are invisible, tasteless, and odorless. When cancer manifests, it is impossible to determine precisely its etiology or cause, but there is a large literature proving that radiation causes cancer, including the data from Hiroshima and Nagasaki.

Here are descriptions of just five of the radioactive elements that are continually being released into the air and water at Fukushima:

- **Tritium** is radioactive hydrogen ^3H. There is no way of separating tritium from contaminated water as it combines with oxygen to form HTO. The only known material that can prevent the escape of tritium is gold, because it is so dense, so all reactors continuously emit large quantities of tritium into the air and cooling water as they operate. Tritium concentrates in aquatic organisms including algae, seaweed, crustaceans, and fish, and also in terrestrial food. Like all radioactive elements, it is tasteless, odorless, and invisible, and will therefore inevitably be inhaled or ingested through food. It passes unhindered through the skin and lungs if a person is immersed in fog containing tritiated water near a reactor. It can cause brain tumors, birth deformities, and cancer in many organs. Tritium has a half-life of

12.3 years—meaning that in 12.3 years, one-half of
its radioactive energy will have decayed—so it remains radioactive for over one hundred years.

- **Cesium-137** is a beta and high-energy gamma
  emitter with a half-life of thirty years. Cesium is
  detectable as a radioactive hazard for over three
  hundred years. Like all radioactive elements, cesium bio-concentrates at each level of the food chain
  (note: the human body stands atop the food chain).
  As an analogue of potassium, it becomes ubiquitous
  in all cells. Exposure to cesium can induce brain
  cancer, rhabdomyosarcoma (very malignant muscle
  tumors), ovarian or testicular cancer, and genetic
  disease.

- **Strontium-90** is a high-energy beta emitter with
  a half-life of twenty-eight years. As a calcium analogue, it is a bone seeker. It concentrates in the food
  chain, specifically milk (including breast milk), and
  is laid down in bones and teeth in the human body.
  Exposure to strontium-90 can lead to carcinomas of
  the breast and bone and to leukemia.

- **Radioactive iodine-131** is a beta and gamma emitter with a half-life of eight days. It remains hazardous for ten weeks. It bioconcentrates in the food
  chain: first in vegetables and milk, then the human
  thyroid gland, where it is a potent carcinogen inducing thyroid disease and/or thyroid cancer. It is
  important to note that of 295,211 children under

the age of eighteen who have been examined by thyroid ultrasound in the Fukushima Prefecture, eighty-nine have been diagnosed with thyroid cancer and forty-two more are suspected to have the disease.[5] In Chornobyl, thyroid cancers were not diagnosed until four years after the accident. This early manifestation at Fukushima indicates that the Japanese children almost certainly received a high dose of radioactive iodine, and along with iodine, high doses of many other isotopes. Obviously, the exposed population will have been similarly contaminated so the rate of other types of cancer is almost certain to rise.

- **Plutonium**, one of the most deadly elements, is an alpha emitter. It is highly toxic, and one millionth of a gram will induce cancer if inhaled into the lungs. As an iron analogue, it combines with the iron-transferring protein transferrin, and it causes liver cancer, bone cancer, leukemia, and multiple myeloma. Plutonium concentrates in the testicles and ovaries, where it can induce testicular or ovarian cancer and genetic diseases in future generations. It is also teratogenic, killing cells in a developing fetus to cause severe congenital abnormalities. As a result of plutonium exposure from Chornobyl, there are medical homes full of children with deformities never before seen in the history of medicine. The half-life of plutonium is 24,400 years, and thus it is radioactive for approximately 250,000 years. Plutonium is also fuel for atomic bombs. Five kilograms is enough fuel for a weapon that would vaporize a city. Each reactor makes 250 kilograms of plutonium a year. It is postulated that less than one kilogram of plutonium, if adequately distributed, could induce lung cancer in every person on earth.

The radioactive contamination and fallout from nuclear power plant accidents will have serious long-term medical ramifications because the released radioactive elements will continue to concentrate in food for hundreds to thousands of years, inducing epidemics of cancer, leukemia, and genetic disease. Already we are seeing such pathology and abnormalities in birds and insects. Because they reproduce very fast, it is possible to observe disease caused by radiation over many generations within a relatively short space of time. Pioneering research has demonstrated high rates of tumors, cataracts, genetic mutations, sterility, and reduced brain size among birds in the exclusion zones of both Chornobyl and Fukushima. What happens to animals will happen to human beings.[6]

The Japanese government is desperately trying to clean up the radioactive contamination from Fukushima Daiichi. But in reality, all that can be done is to collect it, place it in containers—usually plastic bags—and transfer it to an-

other location. Some contractors have allowed their workers to empty radioactive debris, soil, and leaves into streams
and other illegal places. We do not know how to neutralize
these elements nor how to prevent them from spreading in
the future. The main question becomes where to store the
contaminated material safely away from the environment for
thousands of years. No container remains effective for longer
than one hundred years. Sooner or later, they will leak long-
lived radioactive elements. There is no safe place in Japan
to store this amount of radioactive soil and water, let alone
the thousands of tons of accumulated high-level radioactive
waste at the fifty-four nuclear reactors in Japan.

Cancer, congenital anomalies, contaminated food—this is
the legacy we leave to future generations so that we can turn
on our lights and computers whenever we want or make nuclear weapons. It was Einstein who said, "With the unleashed
power of the atom, everything has changed, save our modes
of thinking, and thus we drift toward unparalleled catastrophe." Does the human species have the ability to mature in
time to avert these catastrophes?

In the months and years following the catastrophic nuclear
accident at Fukushima Daiichi, many of the world's major
media representatives and prominent politicians displayed
a woeful ignorance about radiation biology. In response, I
organized a two-day symposium at the New York Academy

of Medicine on March 11 and 12, 2013, on the medical and ecological consequences of Fukushima. I was lucky enough to be able to assemble some of the world's leading scientists, epidemiologists, physicists, and physicians, who presented their latest data and findings relevant to Fukushima. This book, *Crisis Without End*, is a compilation of these important presentations, which contain information that has never before been seen by either the nuclear industry or the public at large.

This book opens with an essay by the former Japanese prime minister Naoto Kan, who was in charge at the time of the accident and who is now an ardent antinuclear advocate. Japanese physicist Dr. Hiroaki Koide writes about the current state of nuclear Japan, and Dr. Hisako Sakiyama, who was a member of the Diet Independent Investigation Committee on risk assessment of low-dose radiation, presents an extremely important report on the committee's findings. Japanese diplomat Akio Matsumura details the failings of the Japanese government and nuclear industry to tell the truth and to keep the population adequately informed about the medical dangers that this dreadful accident imposes both now and in the future.

The data presented by embryologist Dr. Wladimir Wertelecki on the congenital anomalies found in the province of Rivne in the Ukraine after the Chornobyl accident will form the scientific basis on which to understand the epidemiological prognosis of newborn malformations in Japan after Fukushima. In fact, his predictions are now coming to light with reports of an increased incidence of such anomalies now appearing among the irradiated population.

Evolutionary biologist Dr. Timothy Mousseau presents his findings based on the examination of mutations, malformations, and tumors among birds, mammals, and insects within the exclusion zones at Chornobyl and Fukushima. The effect of radiation on the biological systems of mammals, birds, and insects is directly applicable to human health, and his pioneering work on internal emitters and "low-dose radiation" will change any notions of safe radiation exposure promoted by the nuclear industry and its allied bodies—the IAEA, the World Health Organization (WHO), the United Nations Scientific Committee on the Effects of Atomic Radiation (UNSCEAR), and the International Commission on Radiological Protection (ICRP).

Epidemiologist Dr. Steven Wing's insightful chapter on the Atomic Bomb Casualty Commission's studies of the Hiroshima and Nagasaki nuclear survivors is also a work of profound importance. This commission failed to study cancer incidence among victims until 1958, thirteen years after the bombs were dropped. They also refrained from collecting data from any of the victims for five years after the dropping of the bombs, which meant that a whole cohort of extremely sensitive individuals died before any mortality or morbidity data could be collected. These flawed studies, taken as gospel by nuclear agencies, form the standard of radiation dose guidelines for the medical and nuclear industry.

Other significant papers include a study by Mary Olson on the variable effects of radiation upon a heterogeneous population of fetuses, children, women, immunosuppressed people, and the aged. Cindy Folkers succinctly outlines the irresponsible absence of regular food testing for radioactive contamination in both Japan and the United States by the EPA, FDA, and other related agencies.

Experienced nuclear engineers David Lochbaum and Arnold Gundersen describe in vivid detail the dynamics of the accident and the nuclear prognostication related to the structurally vulnerable, earthquake-weakened buildings, melted fuel cores, and fuel pools packed with enormous quantities of radioactive waste.

Differing points of view on the biological effects of radiation are covered by Steven Starr, Dr. Ian Fairlie, and Dr. David Brenner. The buildup of high-level radioactive waste in both Japan and the United States is covered by former U.S. Department of Energy official Robert Alvarez and nuclear waste specialist Kevin Kamps. Furthermore, there are provocative and fascinating essays by two giants: David Freeman, former chair of the Tennessee Valley Authority, and Dr. Herbert Abrams, former professor of radiology at Harvard and Stanford and advisor on the BEIR (Biological Effects of Ionizing Radiation) VII report by the National Academy of Sciences.

This volume also includes an outstanding paper by Dr. Alexey Yablokov, who has collated thousands of scientific, medical, and epidemiological papers from the Soviet

Union, the Ukraine, Belarus, and elsewhere, documenting the extraordinary array of diseases and deaths caused by the Chornobyl disaster. Yablokov is a pioneer yet to be adequately recognized by the global scientific community for his extraordinary work.

1

No Nuclear Power Is the Best Nuclear Power

Naoto Kan

The Fukushima nuclear disaster on March 11, 2011, had two causes. The first was the total power outage at the Fukushima Daiichi nuclear power plant due to the massive earthquake and tsunami, both of which were unprecedented in the history of Japan. The second was man-made: no one had anticipated such a scenario, and so the government had not taken precautions to build adequate facilities and communication structures.

On the evening of March 11, approximately eight hours after the earthquake, Unit 1 experienced a meltdown. The melted nuclear fuel accumulated on the floor of the containment vessel, and this was followed by hydrogen explosions at Units 1 through 4 and meltdowns at Units 1, 2, and 3. Around 3 a.m. on March 15, TEPCO, through the Ministry of Economy, Trade, and Industry (METI), requested the evacuation of its workers. If the TEPCO workers had been withdrawn, it would have been almost impossible to keep those nuclear reactors under control. I understood that it would place the TEPCO workers in great danger, but I demanded that they remain there to deal with the nuclear disaster. TEPCO eventually agreed. On March 17, the Self-Defense Forces started dropping water onto the spent-fuel pools from the air. This was my response to the ongoing nuclear disaster.

As the disaster unfolded, I personally reviewed, and had my experts review, the worst-case scenario. There were six nuclear reactors and seven spent-fuel pools at the Fukushima Daiichi nuclear power plant. The Fukushima Daini nuclear power plant, located 7.5 miles from Fukushima Daiichi, had four nuclear reactors and four spent fuel pools. In total, there were ten nuclear reactors and eleven spent fuel pools in the area. Until March 11, the accident at Chornobyl had been the worst nuclear disaster in history, but it had involved only one nuclear reactor. In comparison, all ten reactors could have experienced meltdowns and released radioactive materials into the air. If that had happened, it would have been necessary to evacuate an extremely large area. That was what I was most concerned with at the time.

Shunsuke Kondo, then chairman of the Atomic Energy Commission of Japan, pointed out to me that, in the worst-case scenario, people within a radius of 155 miles would have to be evacuated, and they would not be able to return home for ten, twenty, or thirty years. The Tokyo metropolitan area, home to 50 million people and almost half of the entire population of Japan, is within this 155-mile zone. If 50 million people had to abandon their homes, leave their workplaces and their schools, and if patients had to leave their hospitals, there would have been many more victims during the evacuation, and Japan would not have been able to function fully as a nation for a long time. Eventually, through a combination of skillful management and, indeed, divine protection, the spread of radioactivity was minimized by pumping out the reactors before the situation became even more serious. Nevertheless, the worst-case scenario had been dangerously close to becoming a reality.

Japanese nuclear power policy had, until then, been inadequate. Utility companies were not required to prepare for a tsunami by, for example, installing a backup power source at a high elevation. The Nuclear and Industrial Safety Agency (NISA) under METI was the authority that should have played the main role in handling a nuclear power accident. However, its senior members were not nuclear power experts. They were experts in legislation or economic policy. Neither they nor their staff were prepared for a nuclear disaster of this magnitude, which made the disaster even worse than it might have been.

Since 2011, I have thought about how to handle nuclear power plants in the context of domestic and global energy policy. Considering the risk of losing half our land and evacuating half our population, my conclusion is that not having nuclear power plants is the safest energy policy.

When I consider future energy policy, I am reminded that the sun has been the source of almost all energy on Earth for the last 4.5 billion years. When mankind manipulated the atom, paving the way for nuclear power plants as a source of energy, they created a technology that cannot coexist with life on Earth. Future energy policy should instead focus on expanding the use of renewable energy, such as wind, solar, and biomass energy, without recourse to nuclear power or fossil fuels. In Japan, renewable energy is rapidly gaining popularity and we have introduced a feed-in tariff system since the Fukushima disaster.

The risk of accidents is not the only problem with nuclear power plants. They generate spent fuel—nuclear waste—and no viable solution has been found for its safe disposal. Japan has more earthquakes than anywhere else in the world, and it is almost impossible to store nuclear waste safely here for long periods of time. Moreover, the conventional idea that nuclear power is the cheapest source of energy has been fundamentally disproved. Nuclear power is not cheap, especially when reprocessing and waste disposal costs are taken into consideration, and nuclear power plants are not, and never will be, justifiable economically despite what many experts and politicians in Japan still think. Nuclear power is only a transitional and temporary energy source. The technology will not and should not exist in the next century.

2

Living in a Contaminated World

Hiroaki Koide

A nuclear power plant is a facility in which electric power is generated from the energy released by the nuclear fission of uranium. When uranium undergoes fission, fission products accumulate within the core of the reactor. Because the fission products are radioactive, they produce heat.

After Fukushima Daiichi was struck by the earthquake and tsunami, the nuclear power plant lost its ability to generate electricity and to draw electricity from the power grid. The diesel generators for emergency use were flooded by the tsunami. But the radioactive materials in the reactor core continued to produce heat. Without cooling, the reactor core would melt down. Cooling required water, delivering water required a pump, and operating a pump required electricity. But there was no electricity and the pumps were not operable. Nor could anyone deliver water to cool the reactor cores. This could be the fate of any nuclear power plant.

Out of the six nuclear reactors in the Fukushima nuclear power plant, Units 1, 2, and 3 were in operation that day when they were struck by the earthquake and tsunami. Although the operators managed to stop the nuclear fission reaction, they failed to stop the decay heat released by the radioactive materials themselves. This led to meltdowns at Units 1 and 3.

The reactor core consists of around 100 tons of sintered uranium ceramic, which does not melt below 2,800 degrees Celsius. The heat in Unit 1, however, was so intense that its core melted. The section of the reactor that contains the core is like a pressure cooker made out of steel, which melts at 1,400 to 1,500 degrees Celsius. The melted ceramic melted through the steel and onto the floor of the containment vessel, the purpose of which is to seal off radiation. The fuel then burned through the protective wall, and radiation was released into the environment. At the same time, the hydrogen generated when the reactor core melted down caused an explosion in the building.

Cesium-137 was one of the most dangerous radioactive materials to be dispersed by the atomic bomb dropped on Hiroshima. The amount of cesium-137 that was released into the atmosphere by Fukushima Daiichi's Units 1, 2, and 3 was 168 times that of the Hiroshima bomb, according to the Japanese government report to the International Atomic Energy Agency. This is an underestimate. Around 400 to 500 times the amount of cesium-137 dispersed by the

Hiroshima atomic bomb has since been dispersed into the atmosphere due to the accident at Fukushima Daiichi. At the same time, almost the same amount of radioactive material has dissolved into water, flowing into the ground and into the ocean.

The Fukushima nuclear power plant is located on the Pacific coast of the Tohoku Region. To the east is the sea, and when the wind blew from the west, the radiation released from the Fukushima Daiichi nuclear power plant moved over the Pacific Ocean. However, when the wind blew from the south or the north, the radiation moved farther into the Tohoku Region or into the Kanto Region, and if Japanese law had been strictly observed, areas with soil contaminated by over 40,000 becquerels per square meter should have been designated as contaminated. However, altogether, this would have covered an area as large as twenty thousand square kilometers and a vast proportion of the Tohoku and Kanto Regions would have had to be evacuated. Faced with such a reality, the Japanese government decided they could do nothing for the people who lived there, and it abandoned them. More than one hundred thousand people who lived within approximately one thousand square kilometers of the plant were evacuated, losing their homes and now living in exile, but about 10 million people were left in areas that should have been designated as contaminated areas. They continue to be exposed to radiation every day.

The Fukushima Daiichi disaster is ongoing. On March 15,

2011, there was an explosion at Unit 4. Because it was off-line at the time of the disaster, all the fuel rods in the reactor core had been transferred to the spent-fuel pool in the reactor building. There had been 548 fuel assemblies in the core, and the spent-fuel pool held 1,331 fuel assemblies. At the moment, they are at the bottom of the spent-fuel pool. The fuel that sank to the bottom of the pool contains enough cesium-137 to be the equivalent of more than 10,000 Hiroshima atomic bombs. Meanwhile, the reactor building, which was destroyed by the explosion, is still exposed to the environment, and there were aftershocks almost daily in the vicinity of the Fukushima nuclear power plant. If another earthquake occurs and should the spent-fuel pool collapse, it will be impossible to cool.

Japan chose to use nuclear energy. That choice has placed a terrible burden on the nation. It has cast the people living around the nuclear power plant into deep despair. It has forced many workers to engage in a desperate struggle to put an end to the disaster. Unfortunately, the clock cannot be turned back. We live in a contaminated world.

We must do what we can to bring an end to the disaster as soon as possible and to reduce the number of people exposed to radiation—especially children. However, Japan has been using nuclear power generation over a long period of time. Despite those in the political and economic spheres insisting that Japan cannot survive without nuclear power, data clearly show that the power supply would not be affected if Japan were to abolish all of its nuclear power plants. All of the nuclear power plants in Japan should be abolished as soon as possible, and Japan's leaders should guide the nation toward that goal so that an even greater tragedy does not occur.

3

Another Unsurprising Surprise

David Lochbaum

The disaster at Fukushima Daiichi was triggered by a series of foreseeable hazards. The disaster began with an earthquake measuring 9.0 on the Richter scale, which should have come neither as a challenge nor as a surprise. The Fukushima Daiichi plant had been designed for severe accidents, and available evidence suggests that all safety systems survived the shaking and were cooling the reactor core as intended. The earthquake, however, extensively damaged the electric power grid, which the plant needed to power the pumps, the motors, the dampers, the lights, and everything it needed to cool the reactor cores.

It had long been known that the grid was not protected against earthquakes even smaller than 9.0. Forecasting that the grid could fail, workers had installed more than a dozen diesel generators. One diesel generator for each unit was all that was needed to cool the safety systems to prevent reactor core damage. The remaining generators provided backup safety. When the earthquake took away the normal power supply, these emergency diesel generators started automatically, providing power to the equipment needed to cool the reactor cores.

The earthquake, however, also generated a tsunami, which arrived about forty-five minutes later. Forecasting that one day the ocean-side plant might experience a tsunami, the workers had installed a protective seawall around the plant that was nearly fifteen feet tall. Unfortunately, the tsunami that day was nearly forty-five feet tall. Years earlier, researchers in Japan had forecast that the site might be struck by a tsunami close to forty-six feet tall, but the plant's owner and the regulator dismissed this on the grounds that it was overly speculative. No changes were made to the Fukushima seawall. Moreover, the diesel generators for the three reactors operating at the time of the quake were located in the basements of the turbine buildings, which were closest to the waterfront. This placement afforded the greatest protection against the earthquake but the least against flooding. The tsunami, scarcely impeded by the short seawall, inundated the site and flowed into the turbine buildings through open doorways and ventilation system louvers. The diesel generators stopped running as they were submerged in water. The company had put all of its eggs in one soggy basket.

Forecasting that the power grid might be lost and the diesel generators might fail, workers had installed banks of batteries with sufficient capacity to power one safety system for up to eight hours. Some of these were also disabled by the floodwaters, and in any case, the plant was without power for nine days. Forecasting that multiple safety systems might be required, workers had developed backups to the backups, including using diesel-powered pumps on fire trucks and barges to provide cooling water to the reactor cores. But the pressure inside the reactor vessels was nearly four times greater than the water pressure developed by the pumps. In other words, these pumps could not supply makeup water unless the reactor vessel pressure was reduced. Forecasting that it might become necessary to lower the pressure inside the reactor vessel, workers had installed valves that could vent the reactor vessel into the containment building and vent the containment building to the atmosphere, but these valves needed electrical power to work.

Meanwhile, in a cruel irony, the three reactors that were sitting a stone's throw away from the Pacific Ocean faced meltdown due to lack of water to cool them. Forecasting that the reactor cores might overheat and melt down, producing a large amount of hydrogen as the fuel melted, workers had installed systems to purge the air inside the containment building of hydrogen. Even before the plant started up, systems were installed to replace the containment air with nitrogen. The hydrogen released from a damaged quarry reactor core would then mix with the nitrogen. With no oxygen, it could not explode. The accident, however, caused the pressure inside the containment building to rise so high that it forced the hydrogen into the surrounding reactor building, where there was no nitrogen. There were instruments inside the containment building that allowed workers to monitor the amount of hydrogen and the amount of oxygen there, and to vent the containment building when it became necessary. There were, however, no instruments inside the reactor building to monitor hydrogen and oxygen concentrations. Hydrogen gas escaped from the containment buildings into the surrounding reactor buildings, and the result was explosions at three of the reactor buildings.

With all these forecasts, the only surprising thing about Fukushima is that no steps were taken to manage the hazards. The warning signs had been there for many years prior to that disaster.

The three reactor meltdowns forced tens of thousands of people to evacuate their homes, and they are not going back any time soon. The Japan Center for Economic Research recently estimated that the cost of the Fukushima disaster was somewhere between $71 billion and $250 billion. This includes $54 billion to buy the contaminated land from people who had to leave their homes within twenty kilometers of Fukushima Daiichi, and $8 billion in order to compensate the former residents. Even if the actual price tag ends up being on the low end of this $71 billion to $250 billion range, that cost far exceeds the expense of what would have been prudent safety investments years ago.

Had the electrical grid been fortified to withstand an earthquake, the continued availability of electric power would have prevented this disaster. There would have been electrical supplies so that the workers could use the equipment that was already there. Had the seawall been raised to a height taller than a tsunami, the safety equipment would not have been flooded and the combined availability of the normal power supply, the backup power supply, and the backup to the backup power supplies would have prevented this disaster. Had the diesel generators and associated electrical buses been located at various elevations and had there been air-cooled generators that did not require cooling water, the availability of some of this equipment would have prevented this disaster. Had the battery banks been installed such that some of them would have survived the tsunami and the rest of them would have lasted more than eight hours, the disaster would have been averted. Had the Fukushima reactor been equipped with a means to reduce the pressure inside the reactor vessel in the containment so that the diesel-driven fire pumps could have worked, the disaster would have been averted. Had workers been given a viable plan when all those things failed, the disaster would have been averted.

The cost of all of these measures would likely have exceeded $71 billion, but it would not have been necessary to pay for all of them, or even the most expensive of them. All they would have had to do was pay for one of those upgrades, even the cheapest one. Doing nothing against a known hazard is irresponsible, and people should be jailed for those decisions.

All the hazards that factored into Fukushima's tragedy had been predicted many years earlier. Nuclear power plants can be built and can operate successfully. Severe accidents like Fukushima continue to occur because nuclear plant owners continue to pretend that they cannot happen. We can struggle against unknown hazards but we have no excuse for operating plants vulnerable to known hazards. We have the capability to protect against these hazards, and we only need to match our capability with the will to do so. When researchers concluded that Fukushima might experience a tsunami higher than its seawall, it should have led the nuclear plant owners and the regulators to evaluate the need to build a taller seawall and relocate emergency diesel generators, providing a reliable backup. The battery power was designed only to last for eight hours, so somebody should have raised the question of what would happen in the ninth hour. If the answer was "Go back to the drawing board and hope for a miracle," that is the wrong answer. Plant owners and regulators can set lower protective standards than a known hazard as long as there is something other than a miracle to step in to save the day. No one asked the right questions and we are paying a high price for that.

How has Fukushima affected nuclear safety in the United States? Some, including the Nuclear Regulatory Commission (NRC), claim that what happened at Fukushima cannot happen here. They are wrong. Prior to Fukushima, the NRC learned about a plant in South Carolina that could be flooded to a depth of thirteen feet, a foot higher than Fukushima. The NRC's own risk analysis calculated there was a 100 percent chance that one in three reactors at that site would melt down if that occurred. Very little has been done other than hide the documents about this threat.

A hallmark of nuclear safety is defense and depth—a backup to the backup—but we have underestimated the likelihood of a severe accident again and again. There are no nuclear surprises. The only surprise is that we continue to be surprised. We repeat the same actions in the hope of a different result, which is one of the definitions of insanity. This, of course, does not work. The technology is too unforgiving, and had Fukushima aimed higher, we would not be where we are today. More important, tens of thousands of innocent people would be in their homes with their belongings, enjoying undisrupted lives. But that is not the case, and for them and for potentially millions of innocent victims in the future, we must do a better job protecting against known hazards.

4

The Findings of the Diet Independent Investigation Committee

Hisako Sakiyama

Daily life can never return to what it was prior to the Fukushima accident. About 10 percent of our land has been contaminated with more than 9 petabecquerels of radioactive materials from the Daiichi nuclear power plant and more than 150,000 people have been evacuated. The contamination of vegetables, fish, and even drinking water remains a serious concern. The reactor vessels at Fukushima Daiichi are all damaged and continue to release radioactive materials, and there are still 676 tons of spent fuel in the reactor vessels and the cooling pools at Units 1, 2, 3, and 4. The most pressing concern is the cooling pool in Unit 4, which was damaged by a hydrogen explosion and contains more than 200 tons of spent fuel. If it should collapse, the result would be catastrophic.

Japan, a land of earthquakes, has fifty-four nuclear power plants and more than twenty thousand tons of spent fuel, yet until the Fukushima disaster, the majority of Japanese people did not recognize the danger of the situation. One of the reasons for this is that the government and the electric power companies have perpetuated the myth of nuclear safety through the media and through the education system.

The Ministry of Education, Culture Sports, Science, and Technology (MEXT) and electric power companies believed that if people came to suspect that they were exposed to even minute amounts of radiation, it would be difficult for them to promote their nuclear power policy. Prior to March 2011, they distributed textbooks with titles such as *Exciting Nuclear Power Land* and *Challenge! Nuclear Power World* in secondary schools, which taught that nuclear power plants are safe, that power plants are built on hard bedrock, and that they can withstand tsunamis. After the Fukushima accident, the textbooks were recalled.

Nine months after the accident, MEXT distributed new textbooks for primary school and high school students. These had titles such as *Let's Think About Radiation* and *What You Need to Know About Radiation*. Although MEXT claimed that the purpose of these books was to provide students with a basic knowledge of radiation, they only mentioned the accident and the release of radioactive materials in the introduction. They did not provide any information on the amount of radioactivity released by the accident, nor did they provide any maps of the contaminated areas. The guidelines written for the teachers recommended that they create an understanding that there is no clear evidence that radiation levels of lower than 100 millisieverts cause disease.

There is, however, evidence to show that low levels of radiation can cause cancer. It is well established that complex DNA double-strand breaks, which result in error-prone repairs, causing mutations and genomic instability, induce cancer. Even levels as low as 1.3 milligrays can produce double strand breaks, and the number of breaks increases linearly with the dose.

One of the most reliable epidemiological studies is the ongoing Life Span Study (LSS) of atomic bomb survivors, which examined 86,611 atomic bomb survivors. In this study, the average radiation dose was 200 millisieverts with more than 50 percent having a dose lower than 50 millisieverts. The study found that there is no threshold below which there is no risk. Other studies have demonstrated the risks of being exposed to low doses of radiation, including studies examining radiation workers at nuclear facilities and children who have developed leukemia in the vicinity of nuclear power plants. There is evidence, too, that radiation can cause illnesses other than cancer, despite claims by the Japanese government and radiation specialists that the low-level radiation poses no known risks. The dose limit of 20 millisieverts established by the government for the residents of Fukushima Prefecture is therefore endangering people's health, especially the health of infants and children, who are highly susceptible to radiation.

A review of internal conference records at TEPCO and the Federation of Electric Power Companies (FEPC) found that the highest risk for TEPCO was the long-term shutdown of their nuclear reactors, caused by the potential tightening of regulations. TEPCO took the easiest path to avoid this by lobbying the Nuclear Safety Commission (NSC), the Nuclear and Industrial Safety Agency (NISA), and MEXT to relax regulation standards. They succeeded.

FEPC also successfully lobbied radiation specialists, including International Commission on Radiological Protection (ICRP) members and the NSC, to relax radiation protection standards. Unfortunately, many radiation specialists in Japan are obedient subjects of the organizations to which they belong, and one document noted that all FEPC's lobbying demands were reflected in the ICRP's 2007 recommendations. One of the ways the FEPC achieved this was by covering the travel costs for ICRP members attending international conferences. Nevertheless, Japanese ICRP members insist that ICRP is neutral and that it does not represent the interests of the electric power companies. Meanwhile, FEPC tracks radiation research with the intent of promoting only research that will relax radiation regulations.

The diet investigation also revealed that most residents of Fukushima Prefecture did not take any iodine. There were two ways that local mayors received advice as to when residents should take iodine: directly from the NSC, and from the governor of Fukushima Prefecture. The NSC faxed the local Nuclear Emergency Response Headquarters, recommending that residents take iodine, but the fax did not reach the mayors. It disappeared, and to this day nobody knows where it went. The NSC also faxed the Fukushima government, but no one noticed the fax until March 18, after all the residents had evacuated. The governor of Fukushima should have independently advised the residents to take iodine, but he did not do this because he was waiting for advice from the NSC. Some mayors advised people to take iodine; however, many mayors hesitated and did not. Not only were they underinformed, but many were afraid of the side effects that NSC had warned them about and they did not have recourse to medical expertise. The tablets were never distributed to individual homes, and in all, only ten thousand residents ended up taking iodine.

Another issue to emerge from the diet investigation concerned the Radiation Emergency Medicine Network, which was created to provide medical treatment in the event of radiation exposure when an accident occurs and to protect the lives and the health of people under abnormal radiation conditions. Radiation hospitals provide initial medical treatment for all victims. When a primary hospital is unable to treat a patient due to excessive exposure, the patient is transferred to a secondary hospital to measure internal contamination and decontaminate the patient. Where necessary, the patient is transferred to one of only two tertiary hospitals in Japan.

The network was set up without considering the possibility of a large-scale spread of radioactive materials. At the time of the accident there were six primary emergency medical hospitals in Fukushima, of which three were located within a ten-kilometer radius of the power plant. These hospitals became unusable as staff and patients were forced to evacuate. The staff and patients at three other regular hospitals within the zone were also forced to evacuate, and during the course of the evacuation sixty patients died. The diet investigation found that more than 50 percent of the fifty-nine primary hospitals nationwide are located within a twenty-kilometer radius of nuclear power plants, which means they are within the evacuation zone. What is more, the maximum number of patients who can be hospitalized in a primary or secondary hospital is just one or two, while a tertiary hospital can take no more than ten critically ill patients.

Soon after the disaster, Fukushima Prefecture launched a health management survey to investigate the long-term effects of low doses of radiation, some of which has been made public. Thyroid ultrasound examinations were performed on children in Fukushima aged eighteen or younger. In 2011, approximately 38,000 children were examined, and of those children, 186 were found to have a nodule larger than 5 millimeters or a cyst larger than 20 millimeters. Three children were diagnosed with thyroid cancer and seven children were at risk of thyroid cancer. According to Fukushima Medical University's Shunichi Yamashita, who was responsible for the Radiation Medical Science Center's Fukushima Health Management Survey, thyroid cancer is usually found only in one child out of a million, and so it appears that the incidence of thyroid cancer has increased since the accident.

The endless debate on low-dose radiation risks is not a scientific issue but a political, economic, and social issue. Scientists must convey scientific truth; they should not be mouthpieces for governments or power companies. Four reactors at Fukushima are broken and nobody knows how or when they can be isolated from the environment. Since Japan is indeed a land of earthquakes, it is a race against time to shut them down completely. The Japanese government and power companies must make it their priority to stop any further damage and halt the ongoing spread of radioactive substances. It is their responsibility because they promoted nuclear power in the first place. It is also the responsibility of every person in Japan to make sure that all reactors in Japan are shut down. Since September 2013, none of the nuclear power plants has been operating, and with no electricity shortage to speak of, there is no reason that any of them should be restarted.

5

The Contamination of Japan with Radioactive Cesium

Steven Starr

Nuclear technology is the equivalent of acquiring on earth the technology of the heavens. . . . The deployment here on earth of nuclear reactions, a phenomenon occurring naturally only in heavenly bodies and completely unknown to the natural world here on the earth's surface, is . . . a matter of deep significance. For all forms of life, radiation is a threat against which they possess no defense; it is an alien intruder disrupting the principles of life on earth. Our world on the surface of this planet, including life, is composed most basically of chemicals . . . and its cycles take place as processes of combination and dissolution of chemical substances. . . . Nuclear civilization always harbors in its womb a moment of destruction, like a ticking time bomb. The danger it presents . . . is of a kind completely unlike those we have faced before. And now isn't it the case that the ticking of its timer is growing louder and louder in our ears?

—Takagi Jinzaburō, 1986

The destruction of the Fukushima Daiichi nuclear power plant released a huge quantity of highly radioactive isotopes that grossly contaminated the Japanese mainland. Most of these radionuclides had short half-lives, which meant they would self-destruct and disappear in a matter of days or months. But for many of the unfortunate people who inhaled and absorbed these short-lived radioactive poisons, there will be major health consequences.[1]

The disaster also released radionuclides that will not rapidly disappear. These will remain in contaminated Japanese ecosystems, where they will negatively affect the complex life-forms exposed to them. Chief among them is cesium-137,[2] which has taken on special significance because it is the most abundant of the long-lived radionuclides that have persisted in the environment following destruction of the nuclear power plant at Chornobyl.

Cesium-137 has been widely distributed as fallout following catastrophic accidents at nuclear power plants because it is a common fission product that builds up inside the used fuel rods of nuclear reactors, and because it becomes a gas at relatively low temperatures. Any accident that causes the fuel rods to heat to the point of rupture or ignition will cause a large release of highly radioactive cesium gas.[3] Burning fuel rods also release highly radioactive aerosols and "hot particles" into the atmosphere. They are then dispersed by the winds.

Cesium-137 becomes most concentrated in terrestrial ecosystems where it "falls out" or is rained out of the sky, and in this fashion makes its way into waters and soils.[4] Cesium easily moves and spreads in the biosphere, because its most common chemical compounds are highly soluble in water. Consequently, cesium-137 quickly becomes ubiquitous in badly contaminated ecosystems.[5]

Cesium is in the same atomic family as potassium, and it mimics its chemical characteristics. This makes cesium particularly dangerous because it ensures that as a contaminant it will be ingested, since potassium is required by all living things. Cesium is recycled (along with potassium) in soil as a macronutrient, and this process tends to keep cesium in the top soil layers.[6] Scientists now believe that it will be 180 to 320 years before the cesium-137 that contaminated much of Belarus, Ukraine, Russia, and Europe actually disappears from the ecosystems.[7]

INTENSELY RADIOACTIVE FISSION PRODUCTS VERSUS NATURALLY OCCURRING RADIONUCLIDES

Fission products produced by nuclear power plants and weapons, such as cesium-137 and strontium-90, are something new to us as a species. These radionuclides did not exist on Earth in any appreciable quantities during the entire evolution of complex life. Although they are invisible to our senses, they are millions of times more poisonous than most of the common poisons we are familiar with. They cause cancer, leukemia, genetic mutations, birth defects, malformations, and abortions at concentrations almost below human recognition and comprehension. They are lethal at the atomic or molecular level.

These radionuclides emit radiation—invisible forms of matter and energy that we might compare to fire because radiation burns and destroys human tissue. But unlike the fire of fossil fuels, radioactivity cannot be extinguished because it comes from the disintegration of single atoms.

Radioactivity is a term that indicates how many radioactive atoms are disintegrating in a time period. We measure the intensity of radioactivity by the rate of disintegration and the energy this produces. One becquerel equals one atomic disintegration (transformation) per second. One curie, which equals 37 billion becquerels, is defined as the amount of any radioactive material that will decay at a rate of 37 billion disintegrations per second.[8]

Sometimes these man-made radionuclides are compared to naturally occurring radionuclides, such as potassium-40, which is found in bananas and other fruits. But this is a false comparison since most naturally occurring long-lived radioactive elements, commonly found in Earth's crust, are very weakly radioactive.[9] Note that potassium-40 has a specific activity of 71 ten-millionths of a curie per gram. Compare that to 88 curies per gram for cesium-137 and 140 curies per gram for strontium-90.[10]

In other words, cesium-137 is 12 million times more radioactive than potassium-40. This is like comparing an atomic bomb to a stick of dynamite. Another highly radioactive fission product, strontium-90, releases almost 20 million times more radiation per unit mass than potassium-40. Which one of these would you rather have in your bananas?

Current radiation safety exposure standards use mathematical models to calculate the internal "committed" dose of radiation delivered by any given quantity of ionizing radiation. These models average the dose of ionizing radiation over the mass of the organ system or tissue mass where it occurs. This approach essentially ignores—and thus dismisses—the intensity of the given source and instead focuses upon the total amount of radiation released in the tissue.[11] In other words, the models equate the effects of a large amount of diffuse, naturally occurring radiation with that from a small, highly concentrated source as long as they both contain the same total amount of energy. If the total energy in a large bucket of warm water is equivalent to that in a tiny, burning piece of coal, does drinking the warm water have the same biological effect as swallowing the coal?

TOXICITY OF CESIUM-137

The amount of cesium-137 deposited per square kilometer (or square mile) of land defines the degree to which an area is classified as being too radioactive to work or live in. To get an idea of the extreme toxicity of cesium-137, consider how little of it is required to make a large area of land uninhabitable for more than a century.

The lands that were grossly contaminated by the destruction of the Chornobyl nuclear power plant are classified by the number of curies of radiation per square kilometer. Strict radiation-dose control measures were imposed in areas contaminated to levels greater than 15 curies per square kilometer

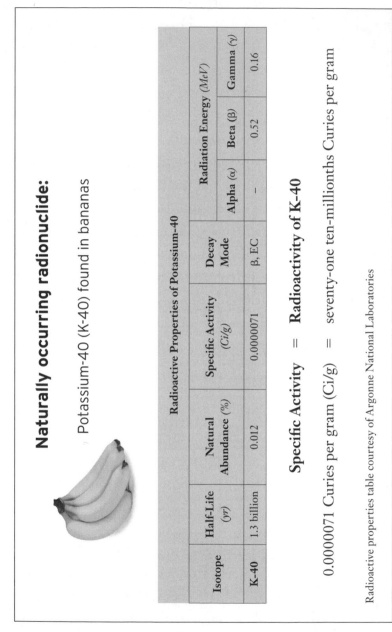

Naturally occurring radionuclide:

Potassium-40 (K-40) found in bananas

Radioactive Properties of Potassium-40

Isotope	Half-Life (yr)	Natural Abundance (%)	Specific Activity (Ci/g)	Decay Mode	Radiation Energy (MeV)		
					Alpha (α)	Beta (β)	Gamma (γ)
K-40	1.3 billion	0.012	0.0000071	β, EC	–	0.52	0.16

Specific Activity = Radioactivity of K-40

0.0000071 Curies per gram (Ci/g) = seventy-one ten-millionths Curies per gram

Radioactive properties table courtesy of Argonne National Laboratories

Figure 5.1. Weakly Radioactive Naturally Occurring Radionuclide

Man-made Radionuclides: Fission Products

Specific Activity = Radioactivity

Radioactive Properties of Key Cesium Isotopes and an Associated Radionuclide

Isotope	Half-Life	Specific Activity (Ci/g)	Decay Mode	Radiation Energy (MeV)		
				Alpha (α)	Beta (β)	Gamma (γ)
Cs-134	2.1 yr	1,300	β	–	0.16	1.6
Cs-135	2.3 million yr	0.0012	β	–	0.067	–
Cs-137	30 yr		β	–	0.19	–

Radioactive Properties of the Key Strontium Isotope and an Associated Radionuclide

Isotope	Half-Life	Specific Activity (Ci/g)	Decay Mode	Radiation Energy (MeV)		
				Alpha (α)	Beta (β)	Gamma (γ)
Sr-90	29 yr	140	β	–	0.20	–

Cesium-137 (CS-137) = 88 curies per gram

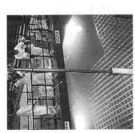

Spent-fuel pool image from U.S. Dept. of Energy

Strontium-90 (Sr-90) = 140 Curies per gram

Radioactive properties table courtesy of Argonne National Laboratories

Figure 5.2

of cesium-137. The total area of this radiation-control zone is huge: 10,000 square kilometers, or 3,861 square miles, which is nearly half the area of the state of New Jersey.[12]

The 1,100-square-mile uninhabitable exclusion zone that surrounds the destroyed Chornobyl reactor has greater than 40 curies of radioactivity per square kilometer, or 104 curies per square mile.

Consider again that one gram of cesium-137 has 88 curies of radioactivity. This means that as little as one-third of a gram of cesium-137, evenly distributed as smoke or a gas over an area of one square kilometer, will make that square kilometer into a radioactive exclusion zone. Less than two grams of cesium-137—a quantity less than half the weight of an American dime—if made a radioactive gas or aerosol and evenly distributed over an area of one square mile, will turn that square mile into a radioactive exclusion zone that will remain uninhabitable for one hundred to two hundred years. For example, the 1,317 square miles of Central Park in New York City can be made uninhabitable for more than a century by less than two grams of cesium-137.

Hard to believe, isn't it? Remember, these nuclear poisons are lethal at the atomic level. There are roughly as many atoms in one gram of cesium-137 (4.39×10^{21} atoms) as there are grains of sand on all the beaches of the world. This means that if one gram of cesium-137 is evenly spread over a square mile, there will be about 1.42 quadrillion (1.42×10^{15}) atoms of cesium-137 per square yard of the contaminated square mile. This works out to about 100,000 disintegrations per second per square yard within this square mile from cesium-137 recently released from a fuel rod inside a destroyed nuclear reactor. The number of atomic disintegrations per second will slowly decrease with time as the cesium-137 self-destructs.

Figure 5.3 illustrates the immense inventories of cesium-137, about 150 million curies, in the form of spent nuclear fuel, located at Indian Point nuclear power plant, which is forty-seven miles from New York City as the radioactive cloud flies. Many of the 104 U.S. commercial nuclear power plants have more than 100 million curies of cesium-137 in their spent-fuel pools. Note that 150 curies of cesium-137 is equal to about 1.7 million grams of cesium-137—a quantity many times greater than that contained within any of the spent pools sitting next to the destroyed reactors at Fukushima Daiichi.

EXTENT OF CESIUM-137 CONTAMINATION OF THE JAPANESE MAINLAND

It is now widely recognized that the nuclear reactors 1, 2, and 3 at Fukushima Daiichi all melted down and melted through their steel reactor vessels within a few days following the earthquake and tsunami of March 11, 2011. This was not made public by either TEPCO or the Japanese government until May 17, 2011, more than two months after the meltdowns and melt-throughs occurred. During these two months, TEPCO continually stated that it was "trying to prevent a meltdown" of the reactors and was not contradicted by Japanese government officials.[13]

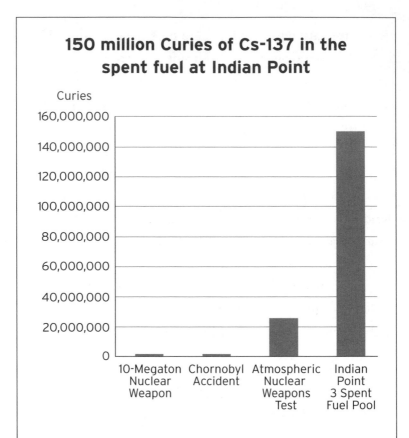

150 million Curies of Cs-137 in the spent fuel at Indian Point

Sources: Reconstruction and Analysis of Cesium-137 Fallout Deposition Patterns in the Marshall Islands, U.S. Centers for Disease Control, 200; National Council on Radiation Protection and Measurement, Cesium-137 in the Environment, Report No. 154, September 2007, Table 3.1,; Nuclear Energy Institute, Spent Nuclear Fuel as U.S. Reactors, December 2011,; and U.S. NRC, Characteristics for the Representative Commercial Spent Fuel Assembly for Preclosure Normal Operations, May 2007, Table 16.

Figure 5.3

The greatest amounts of highly radioactive gases and aerosols were released shortly after the meltdowns occurred. Approximately 80 percent of the radioactive material initially released by the reactors is believed to have traveled away from Japan, over the Pacific. However, the remaining 20 percent was dispersed over the Japanese mainland.

On March 11, the U.S. National Nuclear Security Administration offered the use of its NA-42 Aerial Measuring System to the Japanese government, and the National Atmospheric Release Advisory Center (NARAC) of the Lawrence Livermore National Laboratory stood up to provide atmospheric modeling projections. With the help of American technical means, Lawrence Livermore was able to produce detailed and timely estimates of the radiation plumes emanating from the destroyed reactors, and presumably these were given to the Japanese government.

Scientists at Lawrence Livermore have published a Power-Point of their computer models that includes a distinct image of the highly radioactive plume from Fukushima blowing south over the Tokyo metropolitan area on March 14, 2011. All the areas that the radioactive plume passed over were contaminated, but it appears that the heaviest contamination was deposited outside the metropolitan area, where rainfall occurred.[14]

Eight months after the disaster, the Japanese science ministry released a map detailing the fallout, which showed that 11,580 square miles (30,000 square kilometers)—equaling 13 percent of the Japanese mainland—had been contaminated with cesium-137. The official map does not indicate any cesium-137 contamination in the Tokyo metropolitan area, unlike an unofficial survey done at about the same time by Professor Yukio Hayakawa of Gunma University.

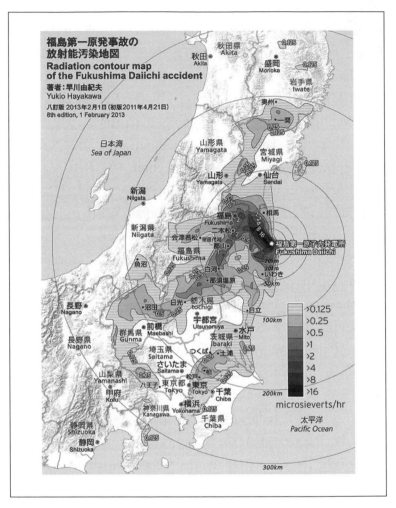

Figure 5.4. Cesium-137 Contamination of Mainland Japan, Including Tokyo

Given the fact that the Japanese government and TEPCO denied for two months that any meltdowns had occurred at Fukushima, one must look at all official data with a healthy degree of skepticism.

The official data admits that 4,500 square miles—an area

almost the size of Connecticut—were found to have radiation levels that exceeded Japan's previously allowable exposure rate of 1 millisievert per year.[15] Rather than evacuate this area, Japan chose to raise its acceptable radiation-exposure rate by twenty times, from 1 millisievert to 20 millisieverts per year.

Although Japan avoided evacuating this large contaminated region, approximately 200 square miles adjacent to the destroyed Fukushima reactors remain so contaminated that they have been declared uninhabitable. More than 160,000 Japanese people were initially evicted from this radioactive "exclusion zone" in May 2011.[16] As of October, some 83,000 still remained homeless, having also lost their property and businesses, and most have received only a small compensation to cover the cost of living as evacuees.[17]

HEALTH RISKS STEMMING FROM INCREASED EXTERNAL AND INTERNAL EXPOSURE TO IONIZING RADIATION

What is the increased health risk to Japanese people based upon their exposure to 20 millisieverts per year? According to the Nuclear Information and Resource Service (NIRS) and Physicians for Social Responsibility (PSR), 20 millisieverts per year is the equivalent of approximately one thousand chest X-rays annually, or three chest X-rays every day of your life. NIRS and PSR state that according to data from the National Academy of Sciences, 20 millisieverts over a lifetime will produce an excess cancer in one in every six people exposed.[18]

Let us also examine figures constructed on the basis of data published by the National Academy of Sciences. In figure 5.5, the vertical Y-axis is calibrated to the number of cancer cases per one hundred thousand age-peers, and the horizontal X-axis depicts the age of the population, beginning at zero years and moving toward old age. Note the allegedly safe dose of twenty millisieverts per year. As a result of this exposure, there will be about one thousand additional cases of cancer in female infants and five hundred cases of cancer in infant boys per one hundred thousand in their age group. There will be an additional one hundred cases of cancer in thirty-year-old males per one hundred thousand in this age peer group.

Children, especially girls, are at the most risk from radiation-induced cancer. In fact, a female infant has a seven times greater risk, and a five-year-old girl has a five times greater risk, of getting a radiation-induced cancer than does a thirty-year-old man. Currently accepted radiation safety standards actually use a "reference man," who is twenty to thirty years of age, as the basis for the standards, which underestimates the dose for infants and children.[19]

There is a great deal of controversy in regards to the accuracy of the methods used to calculate the millisievert, especially the accurate determination of the biological effects of exposure to a source of ionizing radiation that is external to the body versus the long-term internal exposure to the living cells adjacent to radioactive atoms or particles that have been ingested, inhaled, or absorbed by the body.

The risk factors created by the ICRP radiation models were derived largely from studies of Japanese atomic bomb survivors,

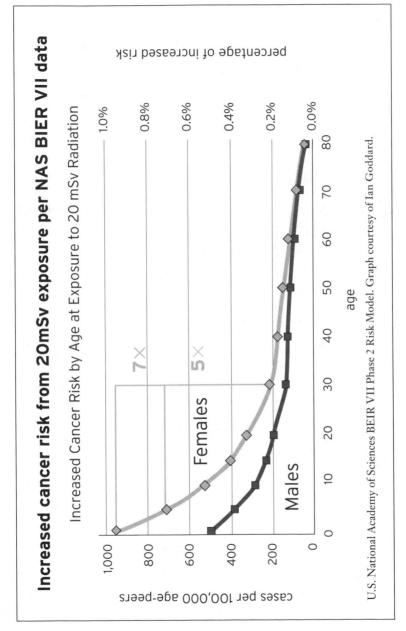

Figure 5.5

who received a homogeneous, high-dose, short external exposure to mainly gamma radiation. The ICRP radiation safety models make the basic assumption that these risk factors can be applied to heterogeneous, low-dose, internal exposure to ionizing radiation. Furthermore, the ICRP standards only cite risks for fatal cancer and include an added element for nonfatal cancer and genetic effects. But noncancer effects from radiation, such as cardiovascular effects, are not included.[20]

The criteria used for determining the evacuation zones was the millisievert (millisievert = one–one thousandth or 0.001 sievert), which is not a measured quantity of radiation, such as the curie or becquerel. Sieverts represent the biological effects of ionizing radiation. A sievert is a derived number, based upon the mathematical models used to convert the measured "absorbed dose" to an "effective," "equivalent," or internal "committed effective dose."[21]

Even the measured absorbed dose includes an important assumption. The absorbed dose averages the amount of energy deposited over a defined mass or volume of tissue, taking no account of the distribution of the energy within the tissue. In other words, the absorbed dose implies that this averaging process will provide sufficient information for the practical application under consideration.[22] It is this approach that equates the "dose" from a weakly radioactive isotope such as potassium-40 with that of an intense radionuclide such as cesium-137. Such a simplistic assumption cannot be made when dealing with biological processes at the atomic and molecular levels.

INCREASED INTERNAL EXPOSURE OF CESIUM-137 THROUGH BIOACCUMULATION AND BIOMAGNIFICATION

In the contaminated land surrounding Chornobyl and Fukushima, the primary route of internal exposure is through the ingestion of foodstuffs contaminated with cesium-137, which tends to bioaccumulate in plants and animals.[23] Cesium-137 has a 110-day biological half-life, meaning that half of it will be excreted from the human body 110 days after it is ingested, inhaled, or absorbed. Like other industrial toxins, cesium-137 often cannot be excreted faster than it is being ingested, so it accumulates and increases its concentration in the plant or animal that is routinely ingesting it.

Cesium-137 also tends to biomagnify as it moves up the food chain. This means it becomes progressively more concentrated in predator species. We have seen this before with other industrial toxins, such as DDT, which can magnify its concentration millions of times from the bottom to the top of a food chain.

Consequently, many of the foodstuffs in a contaminated region tend to contain cesium-137. Those naturally rich in potassium, such as mushrooms and berries, can often have very high concentrations of cesium-137. Dairy products and meats, which come from higher levels of the food chain, will also tend to have higher concentrations.

The International Commission on Radiological Protection (ICRP), which sets radiation safety standards, recognizes that cesium-137 bioaccumulates in humans. Figure 5.6, which comes from the ICRP, compares a single ingestion of

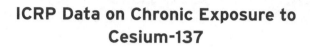

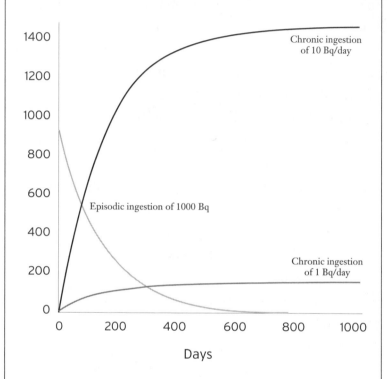

ICRP Data on Chronic Exposure to Cesium-137

Chronic ingestion of 10 Bq/day

Episodic ingestion of 1000 Bq

Chronic ingestion of 1 Bq/day

Days

500 Days' Ingestion of 10 Becquerels per day = total body activity of 1,400 Becquerels

ISSN 0146-6453

Volume 39 No. 3 2009

ISBN 978-0-7020-4191-4

ICRP, 2009, Application of the Commission's Recommendations to the Protection of People Living in Long-term Contaminated Areas After a Nuclear Accident or a Radiation Emergency.
ICRP Publication 111. Ann. ICRP 39 (3)

Figure 5.6

1,000 becquerels of cesium-137, a one-time exposure, with the daily ingestion of 10 becquerels. With the single exposure, note that half the cesium-137 is gone from the body in 110 days.

With the routine, daily ingestion of 10 becquerels of cesium-137, the total radioactivity within the body continues to rise until after about 500 days, when there is a total of more than 1,400 becquerels of radioactivity measured in the body.

Becquerels can be counted in living persons because the decay of cesium-137 leads to the emission of gamma radiation, which passes through the body and can be measured by a whole-body counter. In a 70-kilogram adult, a total-body activity of 1,400 becquerels would correspond to 20 becquerels per kilogram of body weight; in a 20-kilogram child, this same total would represent 70 becquerels per kilogram of body weight. The ICRP does not specify the average age or weight of those examined in the study, but the safety standards that have been set by the nuclear industry do not consider this level of chronic exposure to so-called low-dose radiation to be a significant danger to human health.

The ICRP states in the document that a whole-body activity of 1,400 becquerels is equivalent to an exposure of 0.1 millisieverts per year. The ICRP radiation models, used by radiation health physicists to convert this level of internal absorbed dose to millisieverts, do not predict serious health risks from such exposures. The models predict that it is safe to have ten times this exposure level.[24]

BIOACCUMULATION OF CESIUM-137 IN HUMANS

There is, however, strong evidence that the ingestion of these levels of "low-dose" radiation is, in fact, particularly injurious to infants and children. Research done by Dr. Yuri Bandazhevsky and his colleagues and students in Belarus from 1991 through 1999 correlated whole-body radiation levels of 10 to 30 becquerels per kilogram of whole-body weight with abnormal heart rhythms, and levels of 50 becquerels per kilogram of body weight with irreversible damage to the tissues of the heart and other vital organs. Their findings were first published by a Swiss medical journal in 2003.

One of the key discoveries made by Bandazhevsky was that cesium-137 bioconcentrates in the endocrine and heart tissues, as well as the pancreas, kidneys, and intestines. This finding goes against one of the primary assumptions—that cesium-137 is "distributed uniformly" in human tissues—presently used to calculate millisieverts from internal exposure.

Bandazhevsky's "Chronic Cs-137 Incorporation in Children's Organs"[25] compares the radioactivity measured in thirteen organs of six (autopsied) infants. Very high specific activity—levels of radioactivity up to twenty to forty times higher than in other organs and tissues—was found in the pancreas, thyroid, adrenal glands, thymus, heart, and intestinal walls.

Bandazhevsky summarized his nine years of research in his study "Radioactive Cesium and the Heart." It was never properly translated or publicized, in large part because shortly after Dr. Bandazhevsky presented it to the parliament of Belarus, he was summarily arrested and imprisoned on charges of accepting a bribe. No proof of this, however, was ever produced. Government agents also went to the Gomel State Medical University, where Bandazhevsky was director, and destroyed his archived slides and samples accumulated during nine years of research. Virtually all of the staff who had worked with him on this research were then fired. Some were also prosecuted. Bandazhevsky was replaced with a new director, who denounced Bandazhevsky's work.

After Bandazhevsky was released from prison, he was held under house arrest. It was during this time that he wrote "Radioactive Cesium and the Heart" in an attempt to preserve the findings of his research, knowing that he was likely to soon be imprisoned again for a very long time. He subsequently spent more than four years in a work camp, where he was subjected to torture.[26] Just as Soviet physicians were forbidden to diagnose a radiation-related illness following Chornobyl, the Belarusian government acted to suppress Bandazhevky's work because he had been protesting government efforts to retain and resettle people in the land badly contaminated with cesium-137 (23 percent of Belarus was contaminated by fallout from Chornobyl).

In "Radioactive Cesium and the Heart," Bandazhevsky also correlated the amount of cesium-137 in live children with their heart function. He worked with the BELRAD radiation safety institute, which conducted more than 125,000 whole-body counts on Belarusian children, measuring the amount of internally ingested cesium-137 in each child. From 1996 through 1999, these medical checkups showed that at levels of cesium-137 accumulation over 50 becquerels per kilogram of total body weight, pathological changes in cardiovascular, nervous, endocrine, immune, reproductive, digestive, and excretory systems could be registered.[27]

There were so many contaminated children in Belarus that it was difficult to find any who had not bioaccumulated cesium-137 within their bodies. This indicated just how contaminated the general food supply had become. Figure 5.7 illustrates that only those children with less than 10 becquerels per kilogram of body weight had normal electrocardiograms (ECGs). Thirty-five percent of children with 11 to 37 becquerels per kilogram of their body weight had normal ECGs, 20 percent of children with 37 to 74 becquerels per kilogram of their body weight had normal ECGs, and only 11 percent of those with 74 to 100 becquerels per kilogram of body weight had normal ECGs.

Figure 5.8 illustrates the averaged results from hundreds of human autopsies done during 1997 and is also taken from "Radioactive Cesium and the Heart." Note the very high concentrations of cesium-137 in the thyroid gland. While we generally worry about radioactive iodine concentrating in the thyroid, Bandazhevsky's work shows us that cesium-137 is likely to play a major role in thyroid cancer, too.

I want to point out again that the currently accepted medical and legal understanding of cesium-137 is that it is

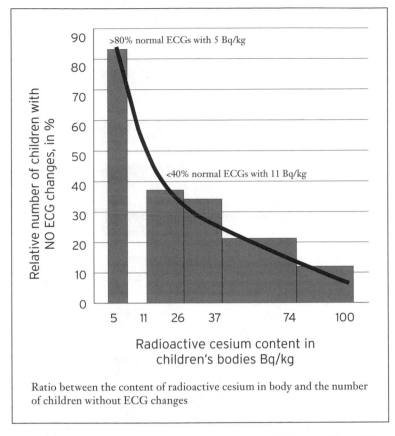

Figure 5.7. Abnormal ECGs in Children with Cesium-137 Greater Than 11 Becquerels Per Kilogram of Total Body Weight from "Radioactive Cesium and the Heart" by Dr. Yuri Bandazhevsky

"distributed fairly uniformly" in human tissues. The autopsied human tissue samples analyzed by Bandazhevsky clearly show that this is not the case. This new understanding needs to be incorporated into the way we understand how internally ingested radionuclides act upon the human body.

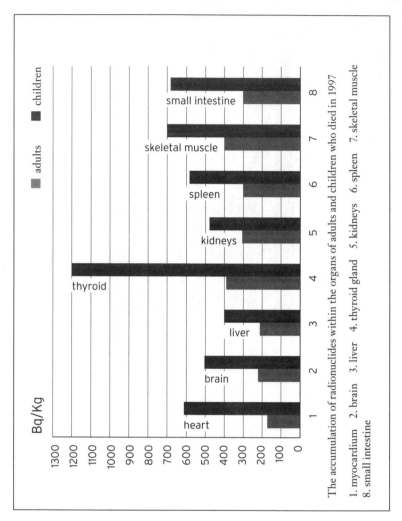

Figure 5.8. Cesium-137 Bioaccumulation in Autopsied Human Tissues from "Radioactive Cesium and the Heart" by Dr. Yuri Bandachevsky

Two million people in Belarus reside on lands severely contaminated by cesium-137. Less than 20 percent of the Belarusian children who live in these contaminated lands are considered to be healthy, although 85 percent to

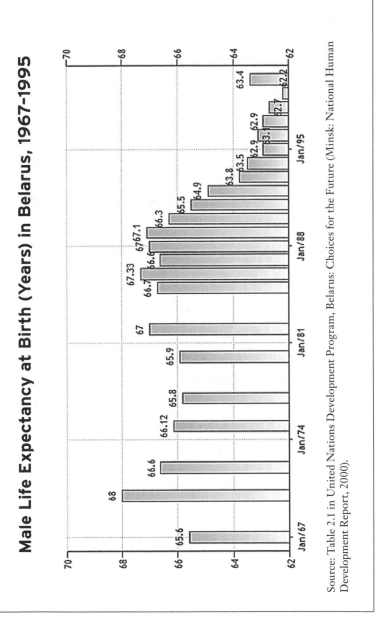

Male Life Expectancy at Birth (Years) in Belarus, 1967–1995

Source: Table 2.1 in United Nations Development Program, Belarus: Choices for the Future (Minsk: National Human Development Report, 2000).

Figure 5.9

90 percent were considered healthy before the nuclear power plant at Chornobyl exploded in 1986.[28] Fourteen years after Chornobyl, 45 percent to 47 percent of high school graduates had physical disorders, including gastrointestinal anomalies, weakened hearts, and cataracts, and 40 percent were diagnosed with chronic "blood disorders" and malfunctioning thyroids.[29] Death rates in Belarus increased dramatically after 1986, while birthrates plummeted.

Twenty-five years after the Chornobyl disaster, the contaminated regions of Ukraine also suffered similar consequences. Dr. Nikolai Omelyanets, deputy head of the National Commission for Radiation Protection in Ukraine, has stated that the population of Ukraine has experienced declining life expectancies and has decreased by 7 million people. In a 2006 interview, Dr. Omelyanets said, "We have found that infant mortality increased 20% to 30% because of chronic exposure to radiation after the accident . . . this information has been ignored by the IAEA and WHO. We sent it to them in March last year and again in June. They've not said why they haven't accepted it."[30]

Dr. Evgenia Stepanova of the Ukrainian government's Research Centre for Radiation Medicine said in 2006: "We're overwhelmed by thyroid cancers, leukemias, and genetic mutations that are not recorded in the WHO data and which were practically unknown twenty years ago."[31] In 2011, Stepanova stated that in the contaminated regions of Ukraine, only 5 to 10 percent of the children are considered to be healthy, while most have a variety of chronic illnesses.

IMPLICATIONS FOR HUMAN HEALTH

The workers exposed to high levels of radiation at the destroyed Fukushima Daiichi nuclear power plant are likely to become severely ill, just as 90 percent of the 830,000 "liquidators" who worked to contain and clean up the Chornobyl disaster did. According to figures given by the Russian authorities, at least 740,000 Chornobyl liquidators became invalids. They aged prematurely, and a higher-than-average number developed various forms of cancer, leukemia, and somatic and neurological psychiatric illnesses. A very large number of them developed cataracts. A significant increase in cancers is to be expected among them in the coming years due to the long latency period of cancer. Independent studies have estimated that 112,000 to 125,000 liquidators died by 2005.[32]

According to the United Nations Scientific Committee on the Effects of Atomic Radiation, between 12,000 and 83,000 children were born with congenital deformations in the region of Chornobyl after the disaster. Only 10 percent of the overall expected damage can be seen in the first generation.[33] In April and May of 2012, there was a significant (51 percent) rise in stillbirths and infant deaths in the four most contaminated prefectures near Fukushima—Miyagi, Gunma, Tochigi, and Ibaraki.

There are many Japanese people now living on lands significantly contaminated with radioactive cesium, where foodstuffs are now being gathered and grown. The massive, ongoing releases of radioactivity into the Pacific Ocean have also widely contaminated the seafood that makes up the traditional Japanese diet. Japanese children living in contaminated regions, who routinely consume contaminated foodstuffs, are at risk for developing the same types of health problems that are often seen in the infants, children, and teenagers of Belarus and Ukraine, who also live in lands contaminated with cesium-137.

It is imperative that we recognize the danger posed to children by the routine ingestion of contaminated foodstuffs. This requires that the currently accepted radiation "safety" standards set up by the nuclear industry, which do not predict any significant health hazards from chronic internal exposure to ionizing radiation, must be either revised or replaced. We need new standards that recognize and predict the dangers to health now manifested in large populations of Belarusian, Ukrainian, and Russian children made sick because they must subsist upon "dirty" foodstuffs contaminated with so-called low-dose radiation.

It is also imperative that we prevent further nuclear disasters that release these fiendishly toxic nuclear poisons into the global ecosystems. Given the immense amounts of long-lived radionuclides that now exist in the used or "spent" nuclear fuel stored at every nuclear power plant, this is an urgent task.

The long-lived radionuclides produced by nuclear power plants are neither "safe" nor "clean." It was and is a very bad idea to routinely manufacture these nuclear poisons simply so we can boil water in order to make steam to generate electricity.[34] It is imperative that we immediately stop nuclear power plants from manufacturing thousands of tons of nuclear poison every year, which create a toxic legacy for the next three thousand generations of human beings.

Most important, we must now turn our full attention to finding a means to safely and permanently remove from the biosphere the more than three hundred thousand tons of high-level nuclear waste that we have already created. These deadly toxins must be isolated from the ecosystems for at least one hundred thousand to one million years. Should we fail to permanently contain and prevent them from entering the biosphere, these nuclear poisons will at some point represent an existential threat to humans and many other forms of complex life.

6

What Did the World Learn from the Fukushima Accident?

Akio Matsumura

I have worked at the United Nations and other international organizations for forty years. I have organized and attended many international conferences, starting with the UN population conference in Bucharest in 1974. Over the years we have discussed in public and in private what you might consider the defining issues of the twenty-first century: population, the environment, socioeconomic issues, disarmament, women and children, and democracy. But we have never discussed how one accident in a nuclear power plant could affect our lives for the next several hundred years, or how we lack a permanent nuclear waste repository that could store spent fuel rods for one hundred thousand years.

I worry about the growing risk to children who continue to be exposed to radiation. Many children will suffer from ill health; many will develop thyroid, lung, and breast cancer. Fukushima has so far emitted more radiation than Chornobyl, and over one million people have died of illness as a result of the Chornobyl accident. In my two visits to

Japan in 2012, I met with political leaders there and asked them for their thoughts on the risk of thyroid cancer in children from the unstable reactors. Few of them knew about the spent fuel rods. Fewer still were thinking about their impact on public health. Undoubtedly some politicians are aware of the potential catastrophe, but even they were surprised when I told them that Unit 4 had ten times more cesium-137 than Chornobyl and five thousand times more than the atomic bomb dropped on Hiroshima seven decades ago. They could not hide their shock when I told them that all of the spent-fuel assemblies at Fukushima Daiichi contained eighty-five times more cesium than Chornobyl, and fifty thousand to one hundred thousand times more than what was released by the bomb dropped on Hiroshima. These same politicians wondered why they had heard none of this from TEPCO.

In April 2012, I met with then–chief cabinet secretary Osamu Fujimura. He assured me he would convey a message to then–prime minister Yoshihiko Noda before he met with U.S. president Barack Obama. Both leaders might have discussed Fukushima at their private meeting, but the idea for an independent assessment team and international aid were not mentioned publicly. This was a mistake. The government's first responsibility is the security of its citizens. Instead of reaching out to independent scientists, they only consulted TEPCO. They focused on minimizing the public-relations fallout instead of the nuclear radiation fallout. In any country, government and industry will not disclose all sensitive information after a disaster, but the secrecy of Japan's leaders has been excessive. Because of the government's unwillingness to share accurate information, the Japanese people must rely on the media for useful information regarding the accident. Unfortunately, journalists in Japan are equally complacent and clueless. There is an astonishing disconnect in Japan between the reality of Fukushima and the fictional image that the public has of what happened there. The media has failed in their job to close this gap. Japanese reporters, with several exceptions, have refused to investigate or ask the right questions about Fukushima.

The government has not made this easy. TEPCO determines when and what information will be released, such as when the reactor site will be open to the media, when video footage of the accident will be released, and whether the accuracy of government medical reports is in question. Without anyone to ask the right questions, the public is left behind a smoke screen and forced to rely on half-truths. The public's efforts to end nuclear power in Japan are inspiring, but they are the result of fear, frustration, and uncertainty. Prime Minister Shinzo Abe will ensure Japan remains dependent on nuclear energy. He will restart Japan's nuclear reactors. Of all the politicians I met, he was the least receptive toward the danger faced by the country's children and the spent fuel rods at Unit 4. It fills me with sadness that we must sacrifice tens of thousands of children for the public to realize disaster is at hand.

I am surprised that one group has not taken forceful action. The Shinto-Buddhist influence on Japanese life has bestowed a sacred importance on the country's natural beauty and resources. Japan's environment has not known a greater threat than that presented by Fukushima. The country's spiritual leaders should be active in reinforcing the country's concern about the ongoing risks.

There have been complete core meltdowns in Units 1, 2, and 3. The Japanese authorities have admitted the possibility that some may have made it through the bottom of the reactor core vessels. It has been speculated that this may lead to unintended criticality resumption of the chain reaction or a powerful steam explosion. Either event could lead to major new releases of radioactivity into the environment.

Units 1 and 3 are sites of particularly intense radiation, making those areas unapproachable. As a result, there have been no moves since the accident to reinforce and repair the structures at those sites. The ability of these structures to withstand a strong earthquake is uncertain.

The temporary cooling pipes installed in each of the crippled reactors pass through debris caused by the accident. They are unprotected and highly vulnerable to damage. Any damage to the pipes could lead to the failure of the cooling system and cause the fuel to overheat. Further fuel damage would lead to the release of radiation, in addition to a possible hydrogen gas explosion and zirconium fire, and fuel melting within the spent-fuel pool.

The frame of the Unit 4 reactor building is seriously damaged. The spent-fuel pool in Unit 4, containing a total of 1,670 tons of fuel, is suspended about 30 meters above the ground. TEPCO plans to remove the spent fuel rods in the coming years, but if there is another massive earthquake nearby, this may not be soon enough. If this pool collapses or drains, the resulting radioactive blast will shut down the entire area.

The plant represents an unprecedented international security risk for human civilization. There is a much higher probability of another disaster than one might think. If there is another earthquake and further meltdowns, our future should not depend on chance, the goodwill of TEPCO, or the Japanese government. Meanwhile, the United States stands silent. It is in U.S. interests to take action. Another disaster could cause high quantities of radiation to reach the West Coast through rain or food. Residents would have to be evacuated and relations within East Asia and with the United States would be strained.

A similar disaster could happen in the United States or elsewhere in the world with a nuclear reactor or temporary spent-fuel storage facilities. There are more than four hundred nuclear power plants operating today—more than one hundred of them in the United States. Several sit near fault lines; others are old. There are also twenty-four temporary spent-fuel facilities holding spent fuel rods like those at Unit 4. Many are only warehouses. Cooling systems are so delicate and prone to failure that something as simple as the corrosion of pipelines can set off a meltdown.

In the case of a nuclear accident in Japan or in any other country you can be sure the reaction of the government and the nuclear power industry will mirror that of Japan after Fukushima. They will control all the information and access to the nuclear power plant site, citing national security concerns. The ability to keep information from the public after a disaster must be a privilege, not an expectation. We need to establish what level of access is necessary for science reporters and what level of government discretion is necessary for national security. We need a framework for this agreement. For now this burden lies with investigators. Even outside disaster scenarios, there is no communication between scientists and politicians. This is true here in the United States too. I was shocked to learn how difficult it has been for a top scientist to contact senators and congressmen. This was not the case twenty years ago. A continuous and open line of communication between independent scientists and journalists and politicians is essential for handling a new nuclear disaster effectively.

International action must be taken. There should be a fact-finding mission to Fukushima comprised of select lawmakers from the United States, Russia, the Ukraine, Germany, the United Kingdom, France, and Canada. Senator Ron Wyden set an example by visiting in 2012. UNICEF and the WHO should establish programs to take measures to save the children who are exposed to radiation in the coming decades. Nuclear scientists and medical doctors should collaborate and develop new technology and medicine to treat illnesses associated with radiation exposure.

When Charles, Prince of Wales, spoke at the Rio+20 conference in 2012, he said with regard to climate change: "It is perhaps a trait of human nature to act only when the worst happens. But that is not a trait we can afford to rely on here." He could have been speaking about Fukushima. Japan is ill equipped to handle the ongoing problem of Fukushima, but this is more than Japan's problem. It has affected and will affect us all.

7

Effects of Ionizing Radiation on Living Systems

David Brenner

We do not know everything we need to know about the impact of low doses of ionizing radiation on the human body. What we do know is that of the main effects of radiation, including its impact on a developing embryo and fetus, the dominant effect in exposed individuals is cancer.

We know about the cancer risks associated with low doses of radiation through studies of the survivors of the atomic bombs that were dropped on Hiroshima and Nagasaki because both events involved large numbers of people and the follow-up, which included more than a hundred thousand individuals, has lasted for a very long time. To understand the carcinogenic effects of low doses of radiation, the follow-up to any study must cover many decades. A single decade is generally insufficient to gain an overall picture.

In Hiroshima, those at the epicenter perished from exposure to extremely high doses of radiation. Between two thousand and three thousand yards away from the epicenter, people were exposed only to low doses of 5 to 100 millisieverts.

This is still higher than the radiation doses at Fukushima. From 1958 to 1998, the total number of solid cancers observed within this group was 4,400. Compare this to the approximately 4,300 expected from a population that was not exposed to additional radiation. The difference is only one hundred, which is a statistically significant increase in cancer risk due to radiation exposure. On the other hand, this is not a large number. In short, low doses of radiation can cause cancer but the individual risks are small.

The reason why an epidemiological study at even lower doses is extremely difficult is that a little more than 40 percent of any population will naturally get cancer, and as you lower the dose of radiation, you have to look for very small increases in risk over and above that 40 percent background. You need larger populations to see that tiny increase in risk. The number of people required for the study is usually prohibitive.

When we talk about small risks, we need to distinguish between risks to individuals (individual risk) and the corresponding public health risks (population risks). For example: suppose there was some activity in which the risk of harm to an individual was one chance in a million. If a small group of people were to take part in that activity, the chance of any harm coming to any one of them would essentially be zero because the numbers are small. In other words, there would basically be no population risk. Now suppose 100 million people were to take part in this same activity. Some of those 100 million people—roughly a hundred people—will definitely be harmed even though the individual risk is exactly the same (one in a million) as it was when only a hundred people were exposed. There is a significant population risk. The bottom line here is that even when the individual risk is very small, the public health significance depends on how many people are exposed to that risk

To link this to the potential effects on human health of the radioactive emissions from the Fukushima Daiichi accident: the risk of dying of radiation-induced cancer among about a million Fukushima residents is roughly one in two thousand—approximately the lifetime risk of dying in Japan from a violent crime. In other words, the individual radiation-associated cancer risks are small. In terms of the population risks, if we take this one-in-two-thousand risk and multiply it by about a million exposed people, a reasonable estimate of the number of people in Fukushima who will ultimately perish from radiation-associated cancer is five hundred.

While the estimated radiation-related risks to individuals are very small, the estimated radiation-related public health consequence—the death of five hundred people—is calamitous. On the other hand, compare that estimate of five hundred deaths with the number of deaths caused by the earthquake and tsunami—approximately eighteen thousand.

As we think about the significance of the Fukushima accident, we need to think about it at two levels: individual risk and population risk. The individual risks, while probably not zero, are very small because the radiation doses are very small. Nevertheless, there is understandably a huge amount of anxiety in Japan focused on individual radiation-related risks. From the perspective of individual risks, there seems to be an imbalance between what we know about the actual individual risks and the level of concern that individuals in Japan have right now about their individual risks.

The relevant concern, in my view, is about the population risks. Considering that the population risk—the worldwide incidence of radiation-related cancer due to the Fukushima accident may well be several thousand—allows one to start posing policy questions about the risks and benefits of nuclear power. We need to seriously address these questions.

We have let the people of Japan down by confusing these two different ways of looking at risk. The individual radiation risks are very small, and so the individual risk for anybody living in Japan or in Fukushima will be small—not zero, but comparable with many other risks that people naturally take in their everyday lives.

We have a responsibility to be more careful about talking about the radiation risks associated with the Fukushima accident. Education is the way to do this. We need to talk to people and explain what the nature of radiation-related risk actually is; we need to explain what we know and what we do not know.

In April 2011, the artists and crew of the Metropolitan Opera in New York City and the American Ballet Theatre were about to embark on tours of Japan. Naturally there was a great deal of concern from everyone about whether they should proceed. I went to the Metropolitan Opera and talked for several hours about what radiation and the risk associated with low doses of radiation are. I tried to be as candid as I could and to express what uncertainties there were. We had an hour of questions, and in the end, the Metropolitan Opera and the American Ballet Theater did go to Japan. If you are willing to sit down and carefully talk to an audience and explain what you know and what you don't know, you can get people to understand what the nature of the risks actually is.

The other part of the story and the reason there is such angst in Japan is the incredible, but not unreasonable, skepticism regarding the information that people are given. Anyone who goes to Japan will see there is such disbelief when it comes to what the authorities are saying about the doses of radiation. We do know what the doses really were—within limits—and we have to reassure people that these were low.

If you could measure everyone's radiation dose directly, you would be able to identify anybody exposed to high doses of radiation. They could then be monitored and treated. It would also reassure the great majority of people who received very low doses or no doses at all. There are many studies to show that if you perform a test, people are more willing to believe the outcome than they are when a person in a white lab coat says, "Don't worry." At Columbia University, we have developed a very high-throughput biodosimetry tool, which is based on the same finger stick that diabetics use. Through this means, we can look at very large populations of, for example, thirty thousand samples a day. In principle, this is one methodology that might reassure people that they are not receiving very high doses and that there is no great conspiracy under way.

At Fukushima there is no doubt that the individual risks are very small, and we must do more to inform and reassure individuals in Fukushima who have been exposed to radiation. Yet there is also no doubt that there will be potentially significant population risks. We therefore need to improve the way we quantify these population risks, because that is the only way we can have a serious conversation about the societal risks and benefits of nuclear power.

8

The Initial Health Effects at Fukushima

Ian Fairlie

On March 11, 2011, following the Great Tohoku Earthquake, a tsunami hit the Fukushima Daiichi nuclear power plant on the east coast of Japan. The resulting surge was over forty feet high at the plant's seawall; it flooded the plant, causing the failures of cooling pumps and diesel electricity generators. During the following days, explosions occurred at Unit 1 on March 12 and at Unit 3 on March 14, which were videotaped and widely broadcast. On March 15, an "explosive event" in Unit 2 was followed by another in the spent-fuel pond of Unit 4 a few minutes later. Finally, on March 16, a major explosion occurred in Unit 4. The latter three explosions were not videotaped because it was dark and the TV crews were not recording at the time.

In sum, three explosions and two explosion-type events destroyed the reactors at Units 1, 2, and 3 and the spent-fuel pool of Unit 4. The spent fuel stored in the pools of all four units overheated as water levels dropped and a fire occurred in the Unit 4 pool. Reactor core meltdowns also occurred in Units 1, 2, and 3. Seven people were killed by the explosions and around 12,000 workers were exposed to more than 250 millisieverts of radiation. Approximately 86,000 people were evacuated from areas near the stricken plant, 76,000 of whom lived within a twenty-kilometer radius. About 8 percent of Japan's surface area was contaminated by the fallout from radioactive plumes emitted by the plant, contaminating food and water.

U.S. military helicopters measured surface levels of cesium-134 and cesium-137 and found plumes of radiation had contaminated some high-population areas, including parts of Tokyo. Even if the approximately 30 million residents of Tokyo received an average of dose of only one millisievert, the resulting population dose of thirty thousand person-sieverts is still a very large collective dose.

Although the accidents at Chornobyl and Fukushima were both catastrophic, the atmospheric bomb tests in the 1950s and 1960s were actually worse in terms of the amounts of radioactivity released into the atmosphere. The fallout from Chornobyl resulted in higher nuclide concentrations over larger land areas compared to that from Fukushima. The highest concentrations were in the Ukraine, Belarus, and the former Soviet Union, but 60 percent of the fallout reached Western Europe, including Britain and France; the latter had unwisely declared that it was beyond the Chornobyl fallout.

In contrast, about 80 percent of the fallout from Fukushima fell on the sea. But the population densities in Japan are much higher than in the Ukraine, Belarus, and the Soviet Union.

Thirty-six petabecquerels (1 petabecquerel = 10^{15} becquerels) of both cesium-134 and cesium-137 were released into the air from Fukushima. Several other estimates—both higher and lower—were made. Japanese estimates, which are perhaps less rigorous, were around 10 petabecquerels.

Larger amounts of radioactive xenon isotopes were emitted from Fukushima than Chornobyl because the accident at Fukushima involved three reactors rather than the one at Chornobyl. These isotopes are noble gases with short half-lives: the longest, xenon-133, has a half-life of 5.2 days.

The February 2013 World Health Organization (WHO) report on Fukushima mentioned that, among those living near Fukushima, there was a 6 percent higher risk of breast cancer in females exposed as infants and a 7 percent higher risk of leukemia in males. These could be underestimates as there were large uncertainties in estimated doses. The report also stated there was a 70 percent higher risk of thyroid cancer in women exposed as infants. Unfortunately, the report was often vague, claiming that health risks for the general population in Japan were "low." It also claimed that there was no discernible increase in health risks expected outside Japan and that one-third of emergency workers at Fukushima Daiichi were expected to have increased risks.

The effects observed after Chornobyl indicate what lies ahead at Fukushima. After about nine months, we can expect the teratogenic, or in utero, effects of radiation exposure, including infant deaths, infant leukemias, and a decline in birth numbers. After two years, we can expect increases in the incidence of leukemia in adults, although this would be hard to detect as leukemia is a relatively rare disease. After four years, we can expect increases in thyroid cancers among women and children. After ten years, there will be increases in the incidence of solid cancers and cardiovascular effects.

Dr. Alfred Körblein, from Nuremberg, Germany, found peaks in infant mortality about six weeks after March 11, 2011. He showed a statistically significant threefold increase in the infant mortality rate: an observed rate of nine per thousand compared to the background rate of three per thousand. This increased infant death rate was clearly anomalous. Nine months later, he observed a 15 percent reduction in live birth numbers in Fukushima Prefecture and a 5 percent reduction in all of Japan, which were also statistically significant. This was similar to what occurred in the city of Kiev nine months after Chornobyl.

Adult leukemia from Chornobyl exposures was difficult to detect because any increases were small compared to existing levels. However, in 2012, Dr. Lydia Zablotska studied over 110,000 Chornobyl liquidators exposed to high levels of radioactivity. She found clear evidence of increases in leukemia, and the results were statistically significant because of the large number of people studied. Also of significance was their finding of a linear dose response down to 115 millisieverts.

In four or five years, there will probably be increases in the incidence of thyroid cancer, although perhaps not to the degree that occurred after Chornobyl. There the affected populations before the accident had iodine deficiencies in their thyroids as they lived thousands of miles from the sea and did not have much seafood in their diets. In Japan, all people live near the sea and most have diets rich in seafood, so their thyroids are stacked up with stable iodine. However, there have already been increases in the number of small cysts and nodules found in children's thyroids in Fukushima, although it remains unclear how many of these will develop into cancers. Thyroid cancers only appeared in children at Chornobyl four years after the accident.

Based on what is known about fallout exposures, estimates can be made of average doses to people and the numbers who will die from cancer from the accident. Once the collective dose to the population is identified, the anticipated number of fatal cancers can be estimated by multiplying the collective dose by the current accepted risk factor of 10 percent per sievert. There have been three studies in this area so far: by the French Institute de Radioprotection et de Sûreté Nucléaire (2011); by Ten Hoeve and Jacobsen (2012) in the United States; and by Beyea, Lyman, and Von Hippel (2013) in the United States. The French study estimated 1,000 to 1,500 deaths, Ten Hoeve and Jacobson 170, and Beyea, Lyman, and Von Hippel about 700. My own study from groundshine (the cesium left on the ground) estimates about 3,000 deaths over the next seventy years, which is how long the cesium will last.

A professor at Hirata Central Hospital studied whole-body counts from internal radiation of 32,000 people who entered his hospital between October 2011 and November 2012. He found a decline in the numbers of people testing positive for internal cesium—from 12 percent in 2011 to 3 percent in 2012. Safecast also has evidence that external radiation levels are declining, albeit slowly. These data are not from TEPCO but from citizen scientists performing their own measurements. These results are slightly encouraging, but clearly tens of thousands of Japanese people, especially in highly contaminated areas, will continue to receive relatively high radiation doses for many decades to come, as is still happening at Chornobyl.

The lesson we should take from Fukushima and Chornobyl is that governments that do not learn from history are condemned to repeat it.

9

The Biological Consequences of Chornobyl and Fukushima

Timothy Mousseau

A number of years ago, prior to March 11, 2011, my colleagues and I worked on the impact of radioactive contaminants in Chornobyl. Our interest was driven by evolutionary ecology and genetics, not radioecology, nor nuclear medicine, nor antinuclear activism. At first, we worked primarily with birds because they were easy to catch, identify, and count. Not discouraged by the fence around Chornobyl, birds entered the most contaminated areas of the site, and tracking them has allowed us to study the long-term health impact of these contaminants.

We have studied biodiversity at Chornobyl since 2000 and Fukushima since 2011. Most organisms that we have examined showed significantly increased rates of genetic damage in direct proportion to the level of exposure to radioactive contaminants. Many organisms showed increased rates of deformities, developmental abnormalities, eye cataracts, and even tumors and cancers. Reduced fertility rates were also common. We found that about 40 percent of male birds in the more contaminated parts of Chornobyl are completely sterile, with no sperm or only a few dead sperm. Many of the birds have reduced life spans. As a consequence, many of these populations are small and have reduced growth rates. Some of these species have actually died out in the most contaminated areas. Individuals of species that are surviving well now may accumulate mutations that will be passed on to the next generation. Some of these individuals live long enough to migrate out of the area, carrying these mutations and their potential effects to populations that have never been exposed to radiation.

Understanding the effects of radioactivity in the environment is not easy. All of us are different. Some of this is the result of genetic mutations that, even if they are expressed (most are not), probably do not influence our survival or ability to reproduce. The natural world is a complicated heterogeneous place. Every point in space and time is slightly different, for instance, with respect to the amount of sunlight it receives, the temperature, the plants and animals that are there, the birds that might fly by. In order to ascertain the effect of radioactivity or radioactive contaminants on an individual, a population, or a species, this variability must be factored into the equation. We have accomplished this by employing a massively replicated biotic inventory design, which involves counting every last organism in hundreds of places in both Chornobyl and Fukushima repeatedly through time.

At Fukushima, as of July 2012, we had made 700 biotic inventories. At Chornobyl, we stopped at 896. We measured the number of birds, the species of birds, the number of spiders, and so forth. We measured many of the environmental variables that might be relevant in determining the presence or absence of a given group of organisms—the meteorology, the hydrology, the species of plants, the presence of water. We set up about half a kilometer of mist nets to catch thousands of birds to obtain blood and feather samples for analysis of their DNA and their overall health. We measured radiation levels, too, first using a very simple measure of radiation levels—the Geiger counter. We then calculated the partial effects of radioactive contaminants on populations while statistically controlling for the many other environmental factors that can influence abundance and diversity. Such an approach had not ever been previously taken by any team of scientists.

We also made use of a radionuclide identifier system to identify the source of radiation in any given area, and we have developed miniature dosimeters using TLDs—tiny crystal chips that capture radiation. By placing a TLD on a bird, releasing the bird, and then recapturing the bird, we can verify how much radiation it is exposed to and accurately estimate the external dose to an individual. We have also measured internal radiation dose by taking birds, putting them in a lead enclosure in the field, and measuring the amount of radioactive material inside their bodies to estimate internal dose. As a result, we have discovered a good relationship between our simple Geiger counter measures of background radiation in a certain location and how much radiation organisms in that same location are experiencing both externally and internally.

There have been, in recent years, a number of reports that the Chornobyl zone is a thriving Eden for wildlife. The origin of this story can be found in a statement released by the Chornobyl Forum of the International Atomic Energy Agency (IAEA) a few years ago, which suggested that the many plant and animal populations had grown and the biome of the Chornobyl exclusion zone had considerably improved because of an absence of humans inside the zone. These statements implied little or no direct effects of radiation on the plants and animals of the region. This report also suggested that much of the human morbidity was a result of stress and other environmental factors unrelated to radiation exposure. But at the time this report was written, there were no rigorous studies of plant and animal biodiversity and abundance in the Chornobyl zone. The absence of data was used to support the argument that radiation effects were largely absent or at least irrelevant for the health of the populations. Much of our recent research into Chornobyl and Fukushima has been inspired by this report. Our goal has been to provide the scientific evidence needed to address these questions thoroughly. As evolutionary biologists, and not antinuclear activists, we had no prior expectations or any interest in any specific outcome.

The Chornobyl exclusion zone is a heterogeneous place. There are vast areas that are free of radioactive contamination. Some of the cleanest areas have less background radiation than Central Park in New York. The background radiation in Central Park is about 0.1 microsievert per hour. In the cleanest parts of the Chornobyl zone, it is about 0.05. The notion that the Chornobyl zone was a new Eden galvanized us to count all the animals there, including the beautiful, endangered Przewalski's horses, which were introduced into the Chornobyl zone following the disaster.

In terms of birds, once we had statistically controlled for other environmental factors, we found that there were only about a third as many birds as there should have been in the highly radioactive areas and only half as many species. Some of the numbers were so low that the populations could not be sustained. Because we noticed that it was difficult to find some insects, we decided to count them, too. One of the most notable discoveries was the near-absence of bees in the most contaminated areas. There were also fewer spiders, fewer grasshoppers, fewer dragonflies, and fewer butterflies (butterflies appear to be hypersensitive to these contaminants, which is consistent with reports in Japan of mutant butterflies post-Fukushima). The same results were found with mammals—from small rodents to deer.

The Ukrainian government has been trying to capitalize on the tourists who want to see the reactor and the wildlife. Unfortunately, there is rarely any wildlife to see, and so they have set up a small zoo in Chornobyl so that tourists, and journalists, can take pictures of wolves and wild boar.

At Fukushima, we compiled three hundred biotic inventories in July 2011 and an additional four hundred inventories in July 2012. We have been working with barn swallows and barn swallow nests, and the overall results have been the same: significantly reduced numbers of individuals in the more contaminated areas. There were fourteen species of birds with which we could perform direct comparisons between Chornobyl and Fukushima, and the relationship between radiation and abundance was found to be about twice as strong in Fukushima in the first year after the disaster as it was in Chornobyl more than twenty years after the disaster. This implies that there is a lack of resistance or an increased radiosensitivity in the Japanese birds. Perhaps some Chornobyl birds have evolved some degree of resistance, or at least the species that are susceptible have significantly declined throughout the exclusion zone over the last twenty-six years. In Chornobyl, every taxonomic group that we examined showed declines in the more contaminated areas, while in Fukushima, only birds, butterflies, and cicadas showed a significant signal of decline. Curiously, the number of spiders actually rose in the more contaminated areas of Fukushima in 2011, perhaps due to reduced numbers of predators (e.g., birds). Based on our extensive surveys of animals in Chornobyl and Fukushima, abundance and diversity in clean areas of the zone may appear to be normal (although this has not been tested), but in areas of significant contamination, many organisms show sufficient declines in abundance to have impacts on overall biodiversity. This refutes the implied positive impacts suggested by the IAEA's Chornobyl Forum reports.

In Chornobyl, we have captured and measured more than two thousand birds over the past few years. We have detected unusual abnormalities among the birds: strange color patterns; patches of white feathers; tumors on beaks, on wings, or around the eye; strange growths on feet or on their rear ends; missing patches of skin; and cataracts in their eyes. Such abnormalities have rarely been reported anywhere else. Chornobyl birds have smaller brains, too. Neurological development was clearly impacted as a consequence of the contamination. Smaller brains mean reduced cognitive function, and the birds are less likely to survive. It remains to be seen what the long-term prospects for wildlife in Fukushima will be. It is still too early to tell, although recent studies on butterflies by Japanese scientists are consistent with our findings for Chornobyl.

It does not take a genius to make the observations we made at Chornobyl and Fukushima, but the problem is that nobody has looked, or if they have looked, they have not followed through by compiling, analyzing, and publishing the data properly in peer-reviewed scientific reports. Unfortunately, there is no funding in this area. Scientists, like plumbers, must be paid for their efforts. My conclusion is that the governments and regulatory bodies associated with nuclear accidents do not want to know the answers to the fundamental questions related to the impact of radiation on wildlife, and by extension, human beings.

10

What the World Health Organization, International Atomic Energy Agency, and International Commission on Radiological Protection Have Falsified

Alexey V. Yablokov

Roughly 35,000 scientific papers have been published on the Chornobyl accident over the past twenty-four years, most of them in a Slavic language. The catastrophe elevated morbidity and mortality in all territories affected by the radioactive fallout. But the official view, based on the IAEA- and WHO-backed Chornobyl Forum (2006), dismissed all the medical and scientific data that did "not correlate with effective doses of irradiation." Their methodology, demanding a statistical correlation between effective doses and mortality/morbidity, was, however, faulty for the following reasons:

1. THE NATURAL PROCESS OF DECAY OF SHORT-LIVED RADIONUCLIDES IS VERY FAST

It is impossible to estimate correctly the average effective dose of radionuclides after an emergency because the natural process of decay of short-lived radionuclides is very

fast. The data for Chornobyl show that the level of ionizing radiation in contaminated areas may change more than
ten thousand times in a year (see figure 10.5). After the
Chornobyl and Fukushima accidents, attention was drawn
to iodine-131, although in some places this radionuclide was
not responsible for the main radiation exposure. Attention
was also drawn to cesium-137, which in some cases was the
source of people's main radiation exposure several months
after the accidents. At the same time, radionuclides such
as barium-140, cesium-136, argentum-110m, cerium-141,
ruthenium-103, strontium-89, zirconium-95, cerium-144,
ruthenium-106, cesium-134, and strontium-90 were hardly
less important, and in sum were probably more important than cesium-137 in forming the ionizing radiation
background in the first few years after Chornobyl in some
areas.

Radionuclide	Activity	Radionuclide	Activity
I-131	223,000	Te-129m	4,000
I-133	48,000	Ru-103	2,880
Te-132	33,000	Mo-99	2,440
Cs-137	11,900	Cs-136	2,740
Cs-134	7,200	Np-239	1,900
Ba-140	7,000	Te-131m	1,700

Source: Sinkko et al., 1987.

Figure 10.1. Surface Air Radiation (mBq/m3) of Some Chornobyl Radionuclides
in Finland on April 28, 1986

2. DOSIMETERS DO NOT DETECT "HOT PARTICLES"

It is impossible to estimate true effective doses because dosimeters do not detect hot particles, which are micron-sized ceramic particles of melting nuclear fuel containing beta and alpha emitters. After Fukushima, they were observed on the West Coast of the United States. Most routine methods of

Radionuclide	Activity	Radionuclide	Activity
Te-132	29,300	Cs-137	5,200
I-132	25,700	Cs-134	2,700
I-131	23,600	Ba-140	2,500
Te-129m	8,000	La-140	2,400
Ru-103	6,100	Mo-99	1,700

Source: Broda, 1987.

Figure 10.2. Concentrations of Chornobyl Radionuclides in 0-5 Centimeter Layer of Soil (Bq/m2) in Krakow, Poland, on May 1, 1986

Radionuclide	Activity	Radionuclide	Activity
Ce-144	63,300	Ce-141	18,000
Pm-144	58,800	Ru-106	14,600
Nb-95	53,650	Cs-137	4,030
Zr-95	35,600	Cs-134	2,000
Ru-103, Rh-103	18,350	La-140	1,100

Source: Grodzinsky, 1995.

Figure 10.3. Radionuclides from Chornobyl (Bq/kg dry weight) in the Leaves of *Aesculus hippocastanum* in Kiev at the End of July 1986

Radionuclide	Activity, Bq	Radionuclide	Activity, Bq
Xe-133	1.1×10^{19}	I-135	2.3×1015
I-131	1.6×10^{17}	Sr-89	2.0×1015
Te-132	8.8×10^{16}	Te-127m	1.1×1015
I-133	4.2×10^{16}	Sr-90	1.4×1014
Cs-134	1.8×10^{16}	Sb-129	1.4×1014
Cs-137	1.5×10^{16}	Np-239	7.6×1013
Sb-127	6.4×10^{15}	Ce-141	1.8×1013
Te-131m	5.0×10^{15}	Zr-95	1.7×1013
Te-129m	3.3×10^{15}	I-132	1.3×1013
Ba-140	3.2×10^{15}	Ce-144	1.1×1013

Source: Japan's Ministry of Economy, Trade and Industry (2011).

Figure 10.4. The Main Radionuclides That Could Have Been Released from the Fukushima Nuclear Power Plant on March 2011

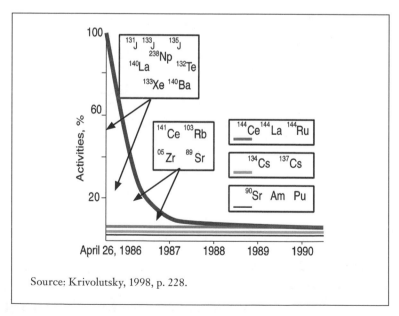

Source: Krivolutsky, 1998, p. 228.

Figure 10.5. Total Chornobyl Radioactivity After April 26, 1986

radiation monitoring do not take into account these particles, but their effect on human radiation exposure can be significant.

3. THE EFFECTS OF EACH RADIONUCLIDE ARE NOT HOMOGENOUS

It is impossible to estimate real effective doses because the effects of each radionuclide are not homogenous in space and time. The vertical migration of radionuclides into the soil causes the level of radiation in the atmosphere to decrease soon after radionuclides are released into an ecosystem. When radionuclides reach root zones (a depth of fifteen to thirty centimeters in the soil), plants bring the radionuclides back to the surface, thus increasing the level of atmosphere ionization for several years. Forest fires, strong winds, and migrating animals can cause horizontal migration, carrying radionuclides for hundreds of kilometers. There are regular daily and seasonal changes in the moisture and density of the top layer of the soil, as well as irregular changes related to precipitation and winds. Because of all of these factors, even at one fixed point, the radiation level may change greatly within hours, days, weeks, and months, making it very difficult—if not impossible—to make any correct calculations of the average external irradiation.

4. THERE ARE TOO MANY VARIABLES TO DETERMINE THE LEVEL OF INTERNAL IRRADIATION BASED ON DIET

The concentration of radionuclides in different kinds of food varies greatly, as does the concentration of radionuclides even

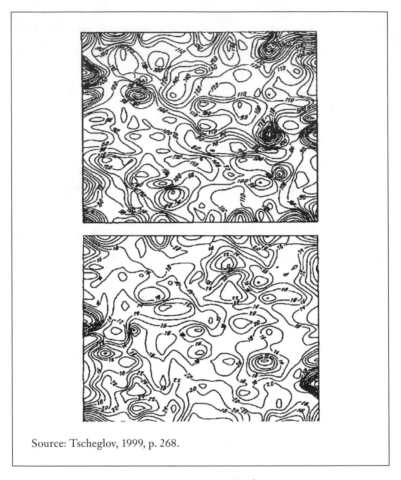

Source: Tscheglov, 1999, p. 268.

Figure 10.6. Pattern of Concentrations (Ci/km^2) of Cesium-137 (top) and Cerium-144 (bottom) in the Soil of the Forest Within Thirty Kilometers of the Chornobyl Nuclear Power Station

in the same foods. There could be variations in the concentrations of radionuclides due to the different ways of treating the same raw food, the coefficients of accumulation of different radionuclides, and differences in individual, seasonal, and local food preferences. Data from Chornobyl and Fukushima have

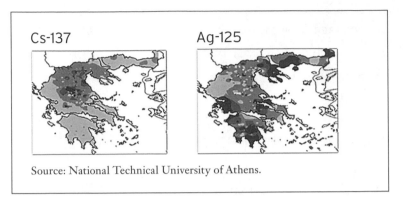

Source: National Technical University of Athens.

Figure 10.7. The Contamination of Greece by Cesium-137 and Argentum-125 from the Chornobyl Fallout

a range of one to two orders of magnitude, which makes calculating an average meaningless. Calculating the average consumption of radionuclides through water and air is less prone to error than through food, but it is also imprecise because of variation in age, gender, body weight, and metabolism. All official dose calculations for the Belarusian people are based on anecdotal data on individual food consumption and behavior (time indoors and outdoors) for 1.1 percent of the irradiated population. It is, without question, nonrepresentative.

5. DIFFERENT PEOPLE HAVE DIFFERENT PERIODS OF RADIONUCLIDE EXCRETION

This depends on a person's physical condition, age, gender, and diet. The average time for excretion of absorbed amounts of radionuclides used in official International Commission on Radiological Protection (ICRP) recommendations for calculating internal irradiation is so simplified that it is meaningless. For instance, according to the ICRP, the average biological half-life of cesium-137 is about seventy days, but in the case of four individuals, it was as varied as one hundred and twenty-four, sixty-one, fifty-four, and thirty-six days.

6. ALL OFFICIAL DOSE ESTIMATIONS NEGLECTED THE EFFECTS OF CERTAIN RADIONUCLIDES

Official dose calculations were based on cesium-137, but in some places, americium-241, plutonium-238 and -240, and strontium-90, which are more difficult to detect, can be the main factors in overall internal and external irradiation.

7. CALCULATIONS USED THE MODEL OF A "CONDITIONAL PERSON"

Until recently, this "conditional person" was a phantom healthy white male, twenty years old and seventy kilograms in weight. The concept of this person is far from scientific and neglects consideration of individual differences as well as age, gender, and ethnic variations in radiosensitivity. Only since 2010 has the ICRP started recommending calculating doses separately for males and women (the male model is known as Golem, the female model Laura), yet they continue to neglect the full spectrum of individual variation.

8. THE DATA IS COMPROMISED

In Chornobyl, as in Fukushima now, much of the data was falsified. In the Soviet Union, medical statistics were secret and were falsified for the first three and a half years after the catastrophe. The official medical data of the hundreds of thousands of liquidators, or cleanup workers, were altered by secret order of the Soviet Ministry of Public Health.

Instead of relying on individual effective equivalent dose, it is possible to rely on much more objective information on the impact of the radionuclide emissions after such nuclear catastrophes as Chornobyl and Fukushima by comparing:

- morbidity/mortality of populations with similar environmental and socioeconomic backgrounds, differing only in the radioactive contamination of their respective territories
- the health of groups of individuals studied year by year after the catastrophe;

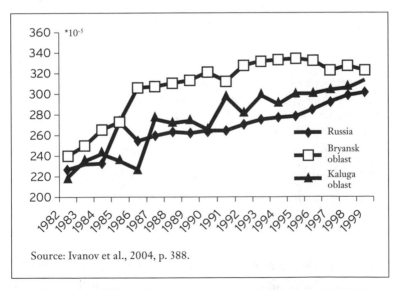

Source: Ivanov et al., 2004, p. 388.

Figure 10.8. Incidence of Solid Cancer in Bryansk Province, Kaluga Province, and Russia

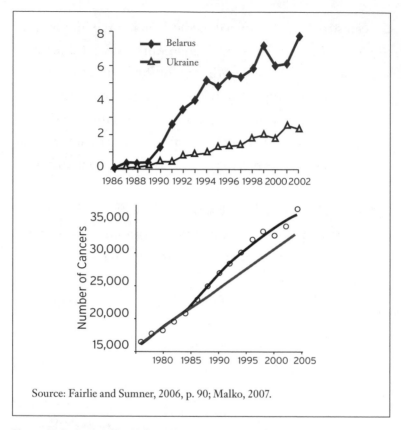

Source: Fairlie and Sumner, 2006, p. 90; Malko, 2007.

Figure 10.9. Cancer Morbidity After Chornobyl: (top) Annual Thyroid Cancer Incidence Rate (Per 100,000) for Persons Who Were Children and Adolescents in 1986; (bottom) the First-Time Registered Cases of All Cancers in Belarus

- the health of individuals in regard to disorders that are historically linked to irradiation, such as stable chromosomal aberrations.

Below are some examples of ways to reveal the real effects of radioactive contamination after Chornobyl. The rise in the cancer rate in contaminated areas (see figures 10.8 and

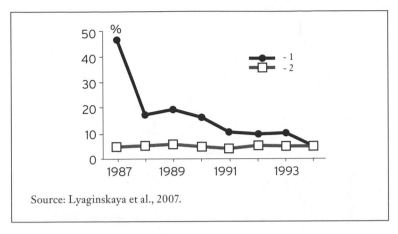

Source: Lyaginskaya et al., 2007.

Figure 10.10. Percent of Miscarriages in Ryazan Province, Russia, from 1987 to 1999: (1) Among Liquidators' Families; (2) Total Population

10.9) is only part of the picture. There are also statistically significant changes over a number of years involving the following:

- prenatal development disorders leading to an increased number of spontaneous abortions (figure 10.10) and premature births
- increase in neonatal, prenatal, and infant mortality (figures 10.11 and 10.12)
- numerous minor and major congenital malformations (figure 10.13)
- lower body weight of newborns
- brain development disorders
- the endocrine system
- the immune system
- premature aging

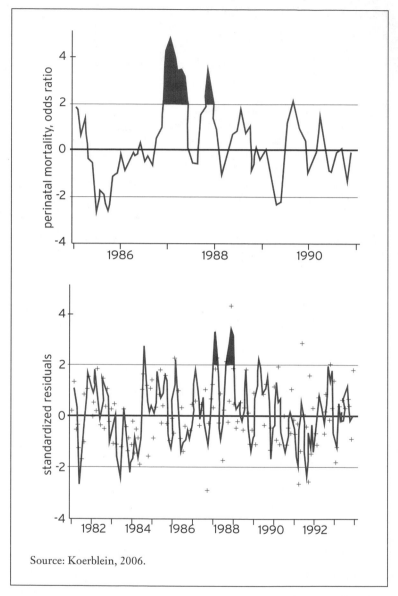

Figure 10.11. Deviation of Infant Mortality from Long-Term Trends in Poland (top) and Germany (bottom)

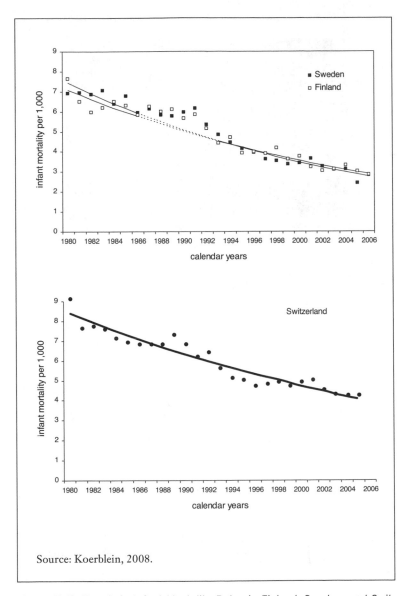

Source: Koerblein, 2008.

Figure 10.12. Trends in Infant Mortality Rates in Finland, Sweden, and Switzerland, from 1980 to 2006, and Undisturbed Trend Line, Based on Official Statistical Data

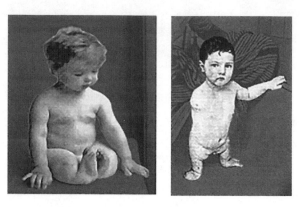

Source: Chornobyl and Nuclear Portal.

Figure 10.13. Some Chornobyl-Induced Congenital Malformations

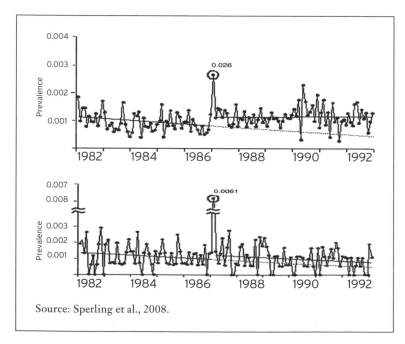

Source: Sperling et al., 2008.

Figure 10.14. Prevalence of Trisomy-21 in Belarus and West Berlin (1982–1992). Change-Point ("Broken Stick") Model.

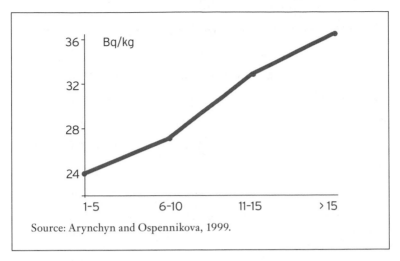

Source: Arynchyn and Ospennikova, 1999.

Figure 10.15 Number of Bilateral Lens Opacities and Level of Incorporated Cesium-137 in Belarusian Children

- somatic and genetic chromosomal mutations and genetic instability (figure 10.14)
- the blood and the circulatory system
- the respiratory system
- the urogenital system
- the skeletal system
- the central nervous system (altering the brain and leading to diminished intelligence and mental disorders)
- the eye (lens) structure (figure 10.15)
- the digestive tract

The radioactive fallout from Chornobyl may also lead to changes in sex ratio: the number of boys born in the Northern Hemisphere decreased by a million after Chornobyl (figure 10.16). There have also been hundreds of examples of health deviations after Chornobyl.

Pro-nuclear scientists often insist that psychological factors ("radiation phobia") are the cause of declining health in radioactive contaminated areas, but morbidity continues to increase even as radiation concerns have decreased. Importantly, voles, swallows, frogs, and pine trees, which do not suffer from radiation phobia, have suffered similar ailments and increased mutation rates.

What will be the total death toll of the Chornobyl catastrophe? The WHO and IAEA only acknowledge the generations spanning 1986 to 2056, with nine thousand people estimated to die from cancer and a further two hundred thousand to fall sick due to the accident—the latter are practically invisible in the total mortality and morbidity of the affected populations. Under pressure, the United Nations Scientific

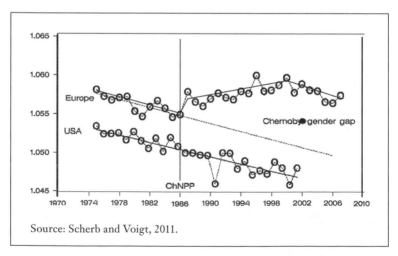

Source: Scherb and Voigt, 2011.

Figure 10.16. The Change in the Sex Ratio Between 1974 and 2006

Committee on the Effects of Atomic Radiation (UNSCEAR) launched discussions on Chornobyl-induced thyroid cancer and autoimmune thyroiditis (which has affected up to several thousand people), leukemia, and cataracts.

Precise calculations based on the official data on mortality in areas contaminated with more than 40 kilobecquerels per square kilometer in six Russian provinces (compared with the neighboring six less contaminated ones) reveal about a 4 percent increase from 1990 to 2004, or nearly 237,000 additional deaths (figure 10.12). About 60 percent of the Chornobyl radionuclides were deposited outside Belarus and Ukraine, and these results indicate that in Europe, Africa, Asia, and even the United States, the total Chornobyl death toll for the period from 1987 to 2004 could reach nearly eight hundred thousand people worldwide. A study, for instance, of the deviation of infant mortality from long-term trends in several European countries shows a spike in infant mortality after the Chornobyl catastrophe (figure 10.13), and there is no explanation for this other than Chornobyl.

The lesson to be learned from Chornobyl is that nuclear electricity brings the same level of risk to humanity and the earth as nuclear weaponry.

11

Congenital Malformations in Rivne, Ukraine

Wladimir Wertelecki

In 2000, our team launched an international program to establish a registry of every child born in the Ukrainian province of Rivne, located two hundred kilometers west of the site of the 1986 Chornobyl accident. The goal was to monitor the population frequency of congenital anomalies. Our team performed ultrasound examinations on nearly 70 percent of pregnant women in Rivne. We reviewed all examinations of stillborn children, and we had newborns examined by trained neonatologists and infants with visible congenital anomalies later monitored by pediatricians and, in most cases, clinical geneticists. We recorded anomalies in children up to the age of one according to methods approved by the Ukrainian Ministry of Health and EUROCAT, a consortium of thirty-eight European systems monitoring congenital anomalies. Our partnership with EUROCAT allowed us to compare congenital malformation rates in Rivne with those elsewhere in Europe. Within two years, it became evident that some congenital anomalies occurred more frequently in northern Rivne-Polissia, henceforth referred to as Polissia.

Polissia is heavily polluted by radiation from the accident at Chornobyl, and there are two additional nuclear power plants of the same age and type as Chornobyl that remain potential sources for further pollution. The area's forested wetlands are geologically different from the fertile plains of southern Rivne, and the soil in Polissia transfers a greater proportion of radioactivity to plants, thereby increasing the quantity of radioactive elements in wood, vegetables, milk, meat, and other products used by the local population. Furthermore, seasonal flooding and frequent forest fires redistribute radioactive materials.

Since 1986, the isolated native population has had no option but to come in contact with radioactive materials. Locally produced milk, cheese, potatoes, and other foods in Polissia are polluted by radioactive elements found in soils. Approximately 67 percent of households burn local wood for cooking or for heating. This wood is a source of radioactive smoke, which is inhaled by both adults and their children. Families also use wood ash to fertilize their home garden plots, further concentrating the radioactive materials as humans and domestic animals consume homegrown vegetables. During harvest, pregnant women are often given easier tasks such as burning dried stems of potato plants containing cesium-137 and strontium-90, which are inhaled as smoke. Consequently, everybody in Polissia has been, and

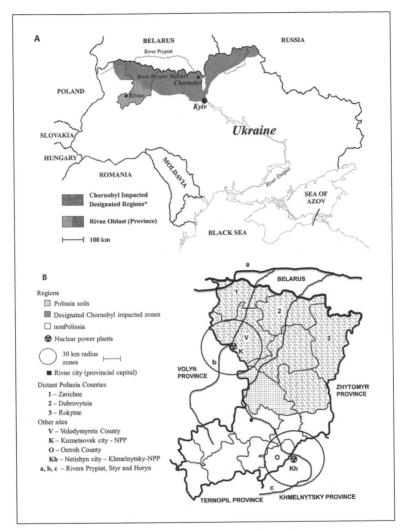

Figure 11.1. Maps of Regions Impacted by Ionizing Radiation from Chornobyl

continues to be, exposed to radiation, with a growing proportion of the population exposed since the moment of their conception by parents who have themselves been exposed to radiation.

Sample	Measurements		
	^{90}Sr, Bq/kg		^{137}Cs, Bq/kg
	Initial	Repeat	
A	43.4 ±17.2	46.8 ±21.4	88.3 ±36.4
B	49.9 ±17.9	32.1 ±24.1	63.6 ±39.3
C	41.3 ±19.9	46.4 ±19.2	24.0 ±22.0
D	82.3 ±21.3	72.2 ±20.0	
E	88.3 ±23.1	84.4 ±28.1	46.1 ±34.6
F	95.6 ±23.1	143.2 ±29.6	
G	327.2 ±86.6	87.3 ±25.1	54.8 ±31.4

Figure 11.2. Radiometry of Dried Potato Stems from Rivne-Polissia Region

When cesium is absorbed by the body, it is excreted in a relatively short time—approximately one year. Strontium, on the other hand, is quickly absorbed by a growing embryo, fetus, and child, and is bound to structures that normally bind calcium, such as bone and teeth, where it can remain for a lifetime.

We determined that an average pregnant woman in Polissia ingests 268 becquerels daily, which is above the upper daily limit of 210 becquerels set for adults by the Soviet Union. The cumulative upper total body count of becquerels for adults was set at 14,800 and for individuals under fifteen was set at 3,700. It is well established that growing organisms are more sensitive to ionizing radiation damage. The upper limit for the rapidly developing human embryo-fetus has yet to be determined.

To simplify the process of estimating radiation exposure and to enhance the accuracy of the estimates, we opted to directly measure whole-body counts of becquerels, which reflect the quantity of cesium-137 incorporated by pregnant women. (Detecting strontium is much harder.) The whole-body count of cesium-137 incorporated by 48 percent of 1,156 pregnant women in Distant Polissia (the three counties farthest north) was above the 3,700-becquerel limit set for individuals under fifteen. Among 6,026 pregnant women investigated, only those from Polissia accumulated significant levels of cesium-137.

	Distant Polissia[a]	Non-Distant Polissia[b]	Non-Polissia[c]
Pregnant Women[d]	1,156	2,534	2,336
Above Bq norm[e] (%)	557 (48.2)	155 (6.1)	3 (0.1)
Children[f]	1,338	3,671	1697
Above Bq norm (%)	162 (12.1)	50 (1.4)	1 (0.1)
Adult Males[f]	2,117	5,885	4,325
Above Bq norm (%)	136 (6.4)	22 (0.4)	-

(a) Includes three most northern counties of Polissia.
(b) Includes four other counties of Polissia.
(c) Includes all other counties except for those in (a) or (b).
(d) Pregnant women seeking prenatal ultrasound examinations at the Rivne Regional Diagnostic Center (2008–2011) who volunteered to undergo the procedure.
(e) Official limits (norms) are 3,700 and 14,800 Bq of cesium-137 for subjects under fifteen years of age and adults, respectively.
(f) 2000–2011 data.

Figure 11.3. Whole Body Counts of Incorporated Cesium-137 Radiation by Rivne Diagnostic Center's Ambulatory Outpatients

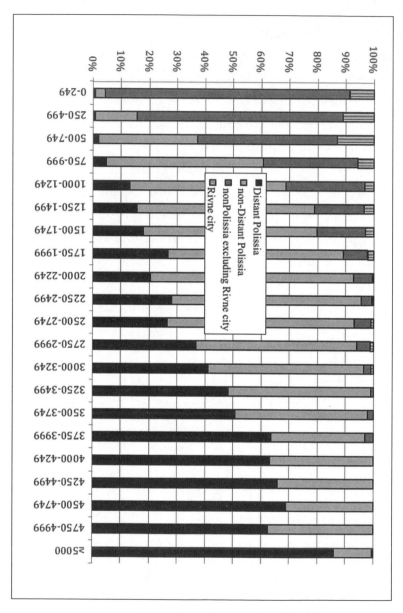

Figure 11.4. Residence and Whole Body Counts (WBC) of Incorporated Ionizing Radiation (Bq 137Cs) Among 9,146 Pregnant Women in Rivne Province (2008-2012)

Area of Residence	Women	AE[1]	OR	P	CL
Polissia	852	13 (1.53)	-	-	-
Non-Polissia	1,417	67 (4.73)	0.31	<0.001	0.16, 0.58
Rivne City	566	36 (6.36)	0.23	<0.001	0.11, 0.45
Khmelnytsky City	1,062	47 (4.43)	0.33	<0.001	0.17, 0.63

Figure 11.5. Alcohol Consumption by Pregnant Women (%)

Category	Polissia	Non-Polissia	Combined
FASD[a]	37[a]	42	79[b]
and Microcephaly[c]	9	11	20
Males	7[e]	6[g]	13
Females	2[f]	5[h]	7
No microcephaly	27	31	58
Males	12	19	31
Females	15	12	27
Gestational age (weeks)[d]			
<35	8	10	18
35–37	9	14	23
≥38	9	6	15
Birth weight (grams)			
<2,500	21	25	46
≥2,500	6	6	12
Prenatal diagnosis	6	6	12

Figure 11.6. All Individuals with Fetal Alcohol Spectrum Disorder (FASD)–Non-Population-Based Observations

The most significant negative impact of radiation on a developing embryo includes anencephaly, which is a developmental deficiency in the skull and in the brain, and microcephaly, which, according to our strict definition, is a reduction in head circumference of three standard deviations below the norm. We found that the frequency of microcephaly was statistically significantly higher in Polissia. We measured the head circumferences of all newborns at birth in one county in Polissia as well as in Rivne City outside Polissia. The head circumferences of the newborns in Polissia were statistically significantly smaller than in Rivne City. We then measured the head circumferences of newborns in another Polissia county and compared these with the head circumferences measured in every county outside Polissia. The results again indicated that head circumferences were statistically significantly reduced in Polissia.

A teratogen is any environmental factor that can cause malformations or developmental alterations. In Ukraine, common teratogens are radiation and alcohol. Both can cause similar congenital anomalies, such as severe or minimal microcephaly. Our program studied not only radiation but also alcohol teratogenicity, partnering with the Collaborative Initiative on Fetal Alcohol Spectrum Disorders (CIFASD), which monitored alcohol use in pregnant women in Rivne and assessed its potential developmental impact on their children. We concluded that alcohol was not a likely cause of higher rates of microcephaly or reduced at-birth head circumferences in Polissia. An analysis of alcohol use by

Incidences and Rates of Neural Anomalies

	Births	Neural Tube Defects	Microcephaly	Microphthalmia
Europe (2000–2008)*	6,392,138	5,860 (9.2)	1,280 (2.0)	486 (0.8)
Rivne (2000–2009)	145,437	303 (20.8)	42 (2.9)	27 (1.9)**
Not impacted by Chornobyl	80,976	138 (17.0)	12 (1.5)	9 (1.1)
Impacted by Chornobyl	64,461	165 (25.6)	30 (4.7)	18 (2.8)**

Rates per 10,000 live births plus stillbirths.

* Data from thirty-one registries (Styria, Austria; Antwerp, Belgium; Hainaut, Belgium; Zagreb, Croatia; Odense, Denmark; Paris, France; Strasbourg, France; Saxony-Anhalt, Germany; Hungary; Cork and Kerry, Ireland; Dublin, Ireland; southeast Ireland; Campania, Italy; Emilia-Romagna, Italy; northeast Italy; Sicily, Italy; Tuscany, Italy; northern Netherlands; Norway; Greater Poland; southern Portugal; Barcelona, Spain; Basque Country, Spain; Vaud, Switzerland; East Midlands and Yorkshire, England; North West Thames, England; northern England; southwest England; Thames Valley, England; Wessex, England; and Wales).
** Excludes three instances of microphthalmia, one in combination with neural tube defects and two in combination with microcephaly.

Figure 11.7

pregnant women clearly shows that alcohol consumption in Polissia is statistically significantly less frequent than outside Polissia.

The range of human congenital anomalies is vast. In Rivne, the rates of sentinel anomalies, such as Down syndrome and cleft lip (with or without associated cleft palate), are well established. The rates of these anomalies in Polissia are similar to the rest of Rivne and to those reported across Europe. On the other hand, the rates of conjoined twins, teratomas, and neural tube defects are elevated in Rivne and even more so in Polissia. The rates of these anomalies in Polissia are among the highest in Europe. Many experts believe that the anomalies are blastopathies, which are anomalies evident in a fertilized ovum (blastula) before it develops into an embryo and it implants in the womb. Recent studies in molecular embryology suggest that any factors that delay the development of a fertilized egg—for instance, radiation damage—may result in the duplication of the axis of an embryo, causing twinning or other blastopathies such as anencephaly. Recent studies also show that female embryos reach developmental stages at a slower pace, which may render them more vulnerable to the kind of blastopathies observed in Rivne.

The Chornobyl accident turned into a catastrophic disaster in great part because of the inadequate response by the Soviet authorities and their chosen experts. These experts, for example, claimed that people in Ukraine who

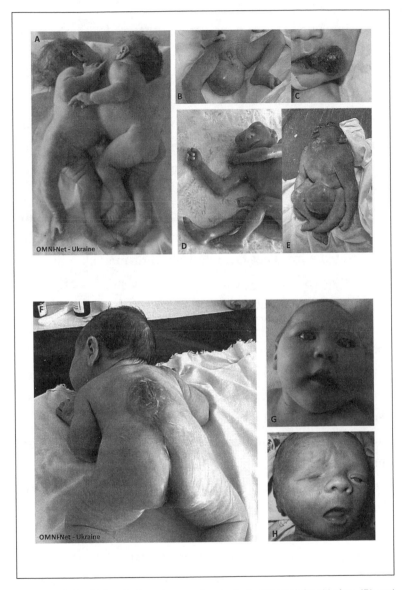

Figure 11.8. Radiation-induced anomalies include (A) conjoined twins, (B) and (C) congenital teratomas, (D) anencephaly, (E) iniencephaly, (F) spina bifida, (G) microcephaly, and (H) microphthalmia.

were impacted by the radiation suffered merely from radiophobia—an abnormal fear of ionizing radiation. Yet evidence of the profound impact of the Chornobyl disaster on Ukrainians can be found in the dramatic drop in the birthrate, which persists even now. The Soviet Union ignored the severe impact of radiation pollution on the population in Polissia—a mistake corrected only in 1991 after Ukraine became independent.

We are aware that reports of elevated rates of congenital anomalies in regions impacted by radiation from Chornobyl are greeted with skepticism and often dismissed. There are many reasons for this, among them the persistent denials by organizations such as the International Atomic Energy Agency (IAEA), the World Health Organization (WHO), and the United Nations Development Programme (UNDP). The IAEA asserts that "because of the relatively low doses to residents of contaminated territories, [there is] no evidence or likelihood of decreased fertility . . . no evidence of any effect on the number of stillbirths, adverse pregnancy outcomes, delivery complications or overall health of children. . . . A modest but steady increase in reported congenital malformations . . . appears related to better reporting, not radiation."

This assertion is not based on actual investigations in areas impacted by Chornobyl but mostly on the results of previous investigations in Hiroshima and Nagasaki, which were sponsored by the Atomic Bomb Casualty Commission

(ABCC). A critical difference between the Hiroshima-Nagasaki and Chornobyl radiation impacts is that radiation exposure from the atomic bombs was external, intense, and short. There was virtually no residual radiation. In contrast, the radiation exposure from Chornobyl was internal, low, and continuous. The impact of radiation on health is cumulative. The average pregnant woman in Polissia absorbs at least 250 becquerels per day, which by the age of twenty-five is equivalent to over 2,200,000 becquerels. A growing number of parents have been exposed to radiation since their own conception.

For the most part, ABCC-sponsored studies were performed before the establishment of the American and later Japanese and European teratology societies, which developed the current criteria for scientific investigations into the human environmental causes of congenital malformations. Launched nearly five years after the bomb blasts, the studies were not based on the exposed population. They were based on children who had not been exposed to radiation but whose parents had been irradiated by the blasts and had survived the explosions and famine that followed.

Two sets of ABCC-sponsored investigations focused on congenital malformations among the children of pregnant women at the time of the blasts. The first involved 205 almost-five-year-old children exposed in utero to the bomb blasts. Clinical examinations without a control group showed that twenty-four (12 percent) had anomalies, including six

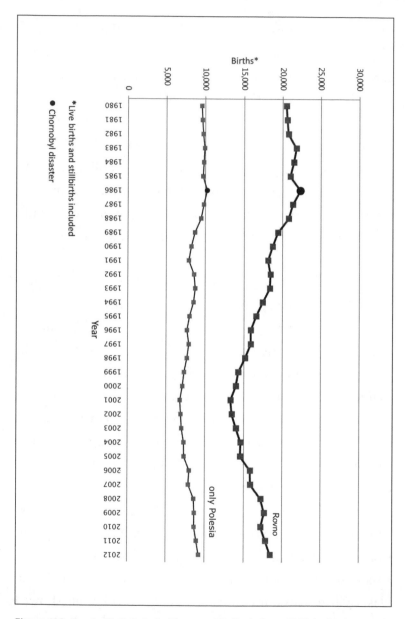

Figure 11.9. Yearly Birth Rate in Rivne and Polissia from 1980 to 2012

(3 percent) instances of microcephaly associated with mental subnormality. Another set of studies focused on mental retardation. They included information on microcephaly but did not focus on congenital malformations. The study group consisted of 1,613 children exposed to the atomic blasts during various states of gestation. Significant effects were evident among those who survived infancy and were exposed at eight to fifteen and sixteen to twenty-five weeks after ovulation, namely, reduction in cognitive function, severe mental retardation, and reduction of head size or obvious microcephaly.

In 1987, it became possible to assign updated dose estimates from a database known as DS86. The analysis estimated a decrease of 25–29 IQ points per gray[1] of uterine absorbed radiation dose. Doses as low as one thousandth of a gray impact the migration of brain neurons. One gray is almost the equivalent of a sievert and a thousandth of a gray, or millisievert, is the unit often used to express safety limits of exposures to radiation. In Europe, the limit for people exposed as part of their occupation is 20 millisieverts per year and 0.3 millisieverts per year for the gonads and uterus respectively. Implicit in these limits is that the gonads and the embryo are at least a hundred times more sensitive to radiation damage than other cells of the adult body. Also implicit is that the exposure is external to the body.

In Polissia, exposure comes through the inhalation and ingestion of radioactive elements, which promptly reach the blood that nourishes the rapidly growing embryonic tissues. It is logical to consider that the high rates of anencephaly, microcephaly, and microphthalmia are likely to be caused by the long-term internal exposure of embryos to low radiation levels in Polissia. This is supported by observations made shortly after the Chornobyl accident. A series of clinical observations indicated a rise in the frequency of congenital malformations, especially anencephaly. Other investigations showed that congenital malformation rates were not elevated among populations residing in regions of Western Europe remote from Chornobyl.

There are two U.S. studies and one British on ionizing radiation exposure from nuclear power plants. The U.S. studies were conducted by the same reputable scientists sponsored by the Centers for Disease Control and Prevention (CDC). Both these studies sought to determine the teratogenic impact of ionizing radiation near the Hanford nuclear complex in Washington State. One study detected higher neural tube defect rates in two counties near the nuclear complex and the other demonstrated higher rates of neural tube defects in parents exposed in their occupation to low levels of radiation. The scientists considered the studies to be sound but rejected the results as "falsely positive conclusions." Among the reasons for this was that the results contradicted those of the ABCC-sponsored studies.

The British study looked at fathers employed at the Sellafield nuclear reprocessing complex in Cumbria in northern England. The results showed a positive association between the total exposure to external ionizing radiation before conception and a higher risk for stillbirths with a congenital anomaly and for stillbirths with neural tube defects.

Two other points deserve attention. In 2013, there were concerns about unusually high rates for neural tube defects in regions close to the Hanford atomic complex, while in northern England and Wales, the frequency of neural tube defects as well as conjoined twins and microcephaly was, after Polissia, among the highest in Europe. The Washington State Department of Health noted twenty-seven confirmed NTD-affected pregnancies from 2010 to 2013 among women residing in a three-county area near Yakima, which is about seventy miles away from the Hanford site. Among the twenty-seven pregnancies, twenty-three were instances of anencephaly, equivalent to a population rate three times higher than the national estimate. This cluster of congenital malformations is under investigation. In Britain, the impact of the Chornobyl radioactive fallout was particularly significant in Cumbria, Wales, and southwest England. The neural tube defects and microcephaly rates in these regions tend to be among the highest in Europe. The central regions of Scandinavia were also heavily impacted by the fallout. Two independent studies, one in Norway and the other in Sweden, showed that individuals most exposed in utero to radiation from Chornobyl demonstrated significant negative impacts on their cerebral functions. These results are consistent with our observations of the reduced head circumferences of newborns in two Polissia counties.

Under the precautionary principle endorsed by medical professionals, those who dictate or advocate policies in the absence of conclusive scientific evidence or consensus have the responsibility to demonstrate that any proposed, imposed, or advocated policies are not harmful to the public or the environment. Official claims that Chornobyl's ionizing radiation is not teratogenic contradict this precautionary principle. Furthermore, the repeated unsubstantiated denial of Chornobyl's teratogenic impact or even potential impact

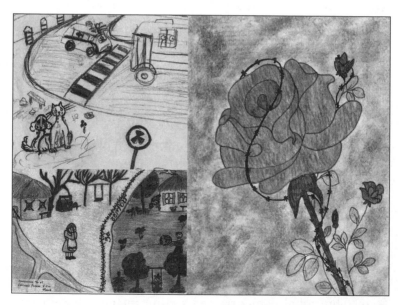

Figure 11.10. As these drawings show, the Chornobyl disaster has had a profound impact on the psyche of children in an elementary school in Ukraine.

discourages attempts to investigate their validity. We hope that through our studies and the events in Fukushima, Japan, will encourage agencies to endorse studies concerned with teratogenic impacts of low-dose ionizing radiation. We also hope that the results of this study provide a starting point for prospective studies of regions impacted by Chornobyl and Fukushima.

12

What Did They Know and When?

Arnold Gundersen

The Fukushima Daiichi accident was made in America. The reactor was designed by General Electric and built by Electric Bond and Share Company (Ebasco). Their engineers made six critical design errors in 1965 that were to doom Japan in 2011:

1. The height of the cliff where the plant was located was reduced from thirty-five meters to ten meters
2. The tsunami wall was too short
3. The diesel generators were placed in the basement
4. The emergency pumps located on the shoreline were not submersible pumps
5. The diesel fuel tanks were placed in the floodplain
6. The flawed Mark I containment was unable to contain the radiation

The first five critical mistakes came from the American engineers' ignorance of the power of a tsunami. Tsunamis, which are produced by a seaquake or underwater volcanic eruption, can travel thousands of miles across open ocean at a speed of 950 kilometers per hour and a height of up to 50 meters. The tsunami that hit Fukushima Daiichi in 2011 was average in size compared to similar waves that had struck the Pacific coast of Japan over the past 120 years. In 1896, the northeastern coast of Japan was hit by a 40-meter tsunami, and in 1933 by a 28-meter tsunami. The 2011 tsunami, however, was only 15 meters high—similar in size to tsunamis in 1923 (13 meters), in 1944 and 1946 (both 12 meters), and in 1954 and 1955 (all of them over 13 meters), just ten years before Fukushima Daiichi was designed. Yet in the face of that history, the engineers at GE and Ebasco reduced the cliff at Daiichi from 35 meters to 10 meters and built a tsunami wall that was only 4 meters high (later raised to 5.7 meters). A tsunami causes the entire ocean to rise. If you are in a boat, you would not notice a tsunami; it is only when it hits a harbor, or the coast, that its terrifying power is revealed. In 2011, the tsunami was 15 meters high and moving at the speed of sound. The wave, when it hit the plant, crested at about 46 meters—higher than all the buildings in the plant.

It is also important to note that not only did the engineers fail to appreciate the magnitude of the tsunami, but GE built the first Mark I reactors on a turnkey contract. They took $60 million for these plants and they lost their shirt. There was enormous pressure on GE to reduce costs because they were losing money dramatically on the dozen reactors they had built on this turnkey process.

In addition, the backup diesel generators were located in the basement with no flood protection and in the path of the rising and surging waters. These were not sealed in waterproof containers and were quickly submerged, rendering them inoperable. There were emergency water pumps located on the shoreline, but they too were flooded, as were the fuel tanks that provided fuel for the generators.

When evaluating the consequences of what happened at Fukushima Daiichi, it is vital to look at a number of assumptions that its designers made. The first assumption was that the containment would maintain its integrity. There are 440 nuclear reactors in the world, and none of them have been designed to handle a detonation shock wave—a wave that travels faster than the speed of sound—because engineers dismissed it as impossible. It did, however, happen. Moreover, there were other serious flaws in the design. Nuclear Regulatory Commission administrator Chuck Casto said "that the Mark I containment is the worst one of all the containments we have," and "in a station blackout, you are going to lose the containment. There is no doubt about it."

Scientists in the United States in 1965 had recognized that the Mark I design had flaws, but the CEO of GE had said that they were "going to ram this nuclear thing through," and ram it through they did. In 1966, GE met with the Atomic Energy Commission's advisory committee on reactor safeguards, which in theory was an independent body designed to protect Americans. Dr. David Okrent, who was on the committee, said that GE made it plain in these meetings that it would not remain in the business of nuclear reactors if it had to redesign its nuclear reactors to better account for core meltdowns—in other words, unless the advisory committee approved the Mark I design. Glenn Seaborg, who was the chairman of the advisory committee at that time, said, "I don't think we have the power to stop them." Indeed, the U.S. government did not have the power to stop GE's faulty design.

About the time the Fukushima Daiichi units were starting up, senior AEC official Dr. Joseph Hendrie wrote that he had serious doubts about the Mark I design, which he believed to be defective and dangerous. He felt they should be eliminated, but he was also aware that in eliminating the Mark I design, "it could well mean the end of nuclear power," which would create "more turmoil than [he] could stand." For forty years, we have known that the Mark I is an accident waiting to happen.

The second assumption that the designers of the reactor made concerned containment leakage. What happened inside the Fukushima Daiichi reactor was that the pressure rose so high that the bolts that held the containment together began to stretch. As a result, it began to leak hot radioactive gases and steam, as well as hydrogen. There were two sources of hydrogen: the zirconium-water reaction created by the fuel, and the meltdown, which brought the fuel into contact with the concrete so that it began to liberate hydrogen. The NRC assumes that containments leak at 1 percent a day. The NRC, however, said on March 23, 2011, that the reactors at Fukushima Daiichi were leaking at 300 percent per day. That means that a volume of gases equivalent to the volume of the containment was being released from the containment and into the environment every eight hours.

The third assumption concerned noble gases, such as xenon and krypton. Nuclear fuel is filled with noble gases, and as long as the fuel maintains its integrity, the gases are trapped inside. During the accident at Fukushima Daiichi, all the noble gases were released. People were breathing in these gases, and the Japanese government had no idea. Data indicate that the concentration of xenon over Chiba Prefecture was 400,000 times normal immediately after the accident—100,000 becquerels per cubic meter for eight days. In other words, in every cubic meter of air over Chiba, there were 1,300 disintegrations emitting radioactivity every second for eight days.

On the ground, there were four radiation detectors that continued to work after the accident. Almost all of them lost power, but a couple of them were battery powered. The normal background level on these radiation detectors was about 0.04 microsieverts. At 5 a.m. on the day after the accident, the radiation around the detectors was ten times the background level. At 6 a.m., it was sixty times the background level. At 9 a.m., it was one hundred and fifty. At 10 a.m., seven hundred. What this means is that somebody in the vicinity of these radiation detectors would have received a yearly dose of radiation in twelve hours. The vents at Fukushima Daiichi were opened after that, so this is a clear indication that the containments were leaking well beforehand. At 3 p.m., these same detectors were measuring thirty thousand times the background level—a yearly dose in ten minutes for the people in Chiba. This was where the detectors were located. It may have been worse elsewhere.

The fourth assumption concerns the decontamination of cesium. The NRC assumes that after a nuclear accident the water inside the torus—the doughnut at the bottom of the containment—removes 99 percent of the cesium. This is a decontamination factor of 100, and it is written into law. It is also said that if the water starts to boil, it is incapable of capturing the cesium and there is no decontamination. Japanese experts claim cesium was captured inside the torus, but the data show that this could not have been the case. Temperatures in the containment were above the boiling point of water, and the flooding had rendered the cooling pumps inoperable. There was no cesium retention inside the torus.

The last assumption concerns hot particles. In February of 2012, I took five samples over the course of five days from the pavements of Tokyo, or in one case a children's park right next to a school. The samples were analyzed by Marco Kaltofen at Worcester Polytechnic. Each of the samples exceeded 7,000 becquerels per milligram, which qualifies as radioactive waste in the United States. Moreover, not only are the residents of Tokyo walking around in radioactive waste, but they are breathing in radioactive material, too. We found this out when we were sent a box of air filters from cars in

Tokyo. Five feet from the box, the Geiger counter started to crackle. Kaltofen took the filters and laid them out on an X-ray plate. After the X-ray plate was left in a safe for several days, there were burn marks on the plate. People were in the cars that carried those filters—children, too. If it is in the air filters, it is in their lungs. We also found cesium on children's shoes. Children tie their shoes; children eat with their hands; this means the cesium is in their stomachs, in their guts, in their intestines.

Three times the volume of noble gases was released at Fukushima Daiichi than at Chornobyl. There were 2.9 petabecquerels of cesium available at Chornobyl; there was almost three times that at Fukushima Daiichi Units 1, 2, and 3. One-third of the cesium was released from Chornobyl. Japanese experts have said only 1 or 2 percent of the cesium was released from Fukushima Daiichi, but that is not the case because the decontamination for cesium was zero.

The one advantage that Fukushima has over Chornobyl is that it is located on the water and for most of the time as the disaster unfolded the wind was blowing out to sea. Nonetheless, about 80 percent of the airborne contamination wound up in the ocean, while the remaining 20 percent, which was at first dispersed in the mountains, was washed into the ocean by rain and snow. Moreover, roughly four hundred tons of groundwater each day is entering through the cracks in the building, where the nuclear fuel remains on the floor. The Japanese are building tanks for this highly contaminated water—one every two and a half days. These tanks are placed in a large tank farm, where they are pumping water from the basements into the seismically unqualified tanks. Liquid releases will continue for years and years into the future. We already know that the liquid releases are ten times those at Chornobyl.

At what point do the risks of a technology become unacceptable? Sooner or later in any foolproof system, the fools are going to exceed the proofs.

13

Management of Spent-Fuel Pools and Radioactive Waste

Robert Alvarez

When I was in the Department of Energy, we looked at a spent-fuel pool problem at the Hanford nuclear site that had been ignored for decades. At the closing briefing we asked what would happen if there was an earthquake and the water drained. There was a hem and haw, and then an old-timer said, "Well, there would be a fire that would make Chornobyl look like a pimple on a pumpkin."

The accident at Fukushima has clearly demonstrated the dangers of spent nuclear fuel storage. Each pool contains irradiated fuel from several years of operations. They contain not one reactor core but several, and there is no secondary barrier of concrete and steel like that which covers the reactor. As a result of the explosions, several pools are now completely open to the atmosphere. The pools of this particular design are more than one hundred feet above the ground, and their structural integrity is now in serious question. They are basically temporary storage structures never intended to hold the quantities they are now holding. Further earthquakes might cause drainage or topple the pools. If they were to drain, there would be a point at which the radiation levels would become so prohibitively high that they would prevent emergency crews from intervening without being exposed to lethal dose rates of five hundred roentgens per hour at fifty to seventy yards. The loss of water could result in overheating from the fuel decay, which could cause melting or an exothermic reaction. The zirconium metal cladding or the metal tubing around the fuel could be set alight, which would result in a large deposit of radioactive material over hundreds of miles.

Irradiated fuel, or spent fuel, is extremely radioactive. An unprotected human one meter away from a single freshly removed spent-fuel assembly would receive a lethal dose of radiation within seconds. This waste contains materials that are radiotoxic, meaning that they create biological damage based on their radioactive properties alone. The U.S. government considers spent nuclear fuel to be one of the most hazardous substances on Earth. This radiotoxic detritus has placed a serious environmental safety and public health burden on our shoulders for tens of thousands of years to come.

The spent-fuel pool at Fukushima Unit 4 contains roughly 37 million curies of cesium-137—about ten times the amount released by the Chornobyl accident. Removing one hundred tons of fuel will not be easy. It is not simply a matter of lifting it out with a crane as if it were cargo on a ship. The basic infrastructure that allows for the safe removal of the spent fuel was destroyed and must be repaired or replaced. All the spent fuel has to be removed underwater with nuclear-safety-rated cranes. It must be transferred into a network of other pools, including a staging pool and an upper pool, which usually remain empty and are required only when moving material in and out. Not only must these pools be repaired, the structural integrity of the building must also be shored up.

Assuming everything proceeded smoothly, it would take time and effort. The rate of transfer of the 1,331 assemblies would be nine or ten assemblies each time. Those assemblies would then be placed in a dry casket—a walled concrete and steel container. Once it is dry, it would be lifted out by a very large crane, placed in a transport facility, and moved to the central pool, which would have to be thinned out to fit the spent fuel and the radioactive ruins.

Pressurized-water reactors do not have elevated pools. Instead, the pools tend to be in buildings adjacent to the reactor. Many of the spent-fuel pool storage areas have cavities underneath them, which could lead to rapid drainage.

Since the early 1980s, the U.S. Nuclear Regulatory Commission (NRC) has approved high-density storage with the expectation that the United States would open a permanent repository for the disposal of spent fuel and defense-level radioactive waste. These pools are now storing four to five times more spent fuel than they were originally designed to hold. The pools were originally intended to be temporary storage facilities for a period of five years and therefore did not require nuclear-safety-rated defense and depth requirements. These pools do not have secondary containments. Some of these pools have buildings with tin roofs—structures you might find at a Costco, a Walmart, or a Ford dealership. They are not required to have redundant power or independent water makeup capability. Only after the Fukushima accident did the Nuclear Regulatory Commission implement requirements that reactor operators have instrumentation in their control rooms to monitor the water levels, water chemistry, and water temperature of the pools. Before that, at some reactors, plant workers had to go and look in the room. There has been at least one occasion when workers did not do this and later discovered that the water level had dropped dramatically.

The spent-fuel pools in the United States contain more spent fuel than in Japan. This is because of indefinite-storage modes, which the nuclear industry has adopted to save money. Furthermore, since the 1990s, U.S. reactor operators are permitted by the NRC to effectively double the amount of time nuclear fuel can be irradiated in a reactor by approving an increase in the percentage of uranium-235, the key fissionable material that generates energy. In doing so, the NRC has bowed to the wishes of nuclear reactor operators, motivated more by economics than spent nuclear fuel storage and disposal. The nuclear power fleet is allowed to operate at the highest burn-up rates in the world. According to engineers from the National Research Council, "the technical basis for the spent fuel currently being discharged and the high-utilization burn-up fuels is not well established. In addition, spent fuel that may have degraded after extended storage may present new obstacles to safe transport."

The reactors operate in turbulent environments. They contain debris. They churn and vibrate, which causes wear and tear on the cladding of the fuel. The cladding, which is only between 0.04 millimeters and 0.08 millimeters thick, becomes thinner and elongated, and the efficient gas pressure inside is two to three times higher. Some types of reactors experience large amounts of grid-to-rod fretting from the high burn-ups.

Spent-fuel pools in the United States are going to run out of room for storage by 2015, which is forcing the nuclear power industry to adopt dry storage but not to thin out their pools. The industry looks as though it will maintain high-density wet storage to the bitter end. It will keep these pools filled to the brim by packing hot spent-fuel assemblies closer together. When there is no longer any room, the industry will start building dry casks.

From the point of view of spent-fuel storage safety, the loss of water is a very serious matter. According to the National Academy of Sciences, due to the enormous decay heat and the reactivity of zirconium, the zirconium cladding can spontaneously combust around eight hundred to one thousand degrees centigrade. It is strongly exothermic and the result could be runaway oxidation that proceeds as a burn front, as in a forest fire or fireworks sparkler.

In 2003, several colleagues and I were stricken from the Christmas card list of many people in the nuclear industry when we published a paper raising concerns about the vulnerability of spent-fuel pools to acts of terror and other events such as earthquakes. We took the literature of the previous twenty-five to thirty years on nuclear spent-fuel safety to the logical extreme. Unhappy with us, the Nuclear Regulatory Commission issued a number of statements and papers in rebuttal. This prompted Congress to ask the National Academy of Sciences to clarify the issue. We went before a special panel, and my colleague Frank von Hippel presented to them what might happen in the case of a pool fire. He illustrated that a pool fire at a commercial nuclear power plant in the United States could be sixty times greater in size than the cordon sanitaire around Chornobyl. We also provided the standard damage estimates that the industry uses to calculate the monetary and carcinogenic estimates. This kind of accident could destabilize and devastate entire nations. The academy agreed with us. They pointed out that these pools are particularly vulnerable to terrorist attacks and that the fires could be significant. The Nuclear Regulatory Commission, however, did nothing to acknowledge the importance of this study.

The Nuclear Regulatory Commission created a workbook involving the San Onofre Nuclear Generating Station. It provides emergency scenarios, such as what would you do if you received a phone call from the staff at San Onofre informing you that they had just had an earthquake, that the roof of the reactor was gone, that the pool was draining, that they had just put a full fresh core in there and the tops of the fuel were already exposed. What might happen? The answer: approximately 86 million curies of the 26 billion curies of radioactivity that would be released into the environment would be cesium-137. Doses within one to ten miles would be anything from prompt lethal to fatal for half of the people (median lethal). From 450 to 5,200 rems is what is known as an ablation dose, which would destroy the thyroid of anyone in a ten-mile radius.

Another exercise concerned a terrorist who has placed a shaped charge on a cask at the Prairie Island Nuclear Generating Plant. What would the release and the doses be? The answer: A cask would release as much as 34,000 curies of radioactivity. Everyone within a ten-mile radius would have a near-lethal if not prompt lethal dose. The reactor is cheek by jowl with the territory of a small Native American tribe. The total effective dose estimate would be 1.9 to 4 rems, while the thyroid dose estimate would be 0.1 to 0.2 rems, which is extremely high. It is also worth noting that within a ten-mile radius of the San Onofre Nuclear Generating Station is the world's largest U.S. Marine Corps base, Camp Pendleton, where there are stationed 64,000 marines and support. This surely has some national security ramifications.

Much has been written and said about Fukushima. What I find interesting is what is not said. There were nine dry casks at the site and they were unscathed by the earthquake and the tsunami. We recommended in 2003 that the spent-fuel pools be returned to their original purpose, which was temporary storage for a five-year period to allow for decay heat before moving them. We suggested that the remaining spent fuel be placed in dry-hardened storage. We estimated it would cost about $3.5 billion to $7 billion and that it would take about ten years. The Electric Power Research Institute estimated it would cost $3.9 billion and that it was prohibitively expensive because the reactor would be out of operation for a while. Even while it was operating, the profits from the reactor were small. My impression is that they treat these reactors as if they were ATM machines. If the consumer were to pay for this, there would be an enormous reduction in potential risks and hazards.

The entire framework for the disposal of high-level radio-active waste, however, is collapsing in the United States. The Yucca Mountain site can no longer be used, and the NRC's attempt to jam as much spent fuel as possible into spent-fuel pools has been rejected by a federal court on the grounds that their assumptions about the consequences of spent-fuel fires had not been tested in a lab. The NRC has now embarked on a very time-consuming environmental impact statement.

Meanwhile, we have a long-term abundance of natural gas, which is making these older single-unit reactors more vulnerable economically. This is placing more pressure on an industry that is more economically motivated than motivated by waste management.

The United States also has about 100 million gallons of military high-level radioactive waste in tanks that are larger than most state capitol domes. Roughly a third of them have leaked. After thirty years, we have spent $120 billion trying to stabilize them, and we have been able to stabilize about 11 percent of the radioactivity. This is a national priority because we must protect rivers such as the Columbia River in the Pacific Northwest and the Savannah River, which supplies drinking water to the southeastern area of the United States.

We have been searching for somewhere to dispose of this toxic waste for close to sixty years, but we need to understand that some of the largest concentrations of artificial radioactivity on the planet are going to remain in storage at U.S. reactors. We have put the disposal cart before the storage horse. We have always thought that we would find a place and there was no need to take the extraordinary steps that nations such as Germany have done to protect their spent fuel. We need a national policy that reduces the hazards presented by these pools and a safe storage policy before we start looking for a geological repository. Storage and stabilization of military high-level waste must also be a national priority. This will be expensive, but the costs of doing too little to fix America's high-level radioactive waste storage vulnerabilities are incalculable.

14

Seventy Years of Radioactive Risks in Japan and America

Kevin Kamps

In August 2010, I was invited on a speaking tour of Japan. My first stops on the tour were Okuma and Futaba, from where I could see the Fukushima Daiichi nuclear plant. From a bluff over the Pacific, I could see the six reactors three and a half miles to the north. Three and a half miles to the south, I could see the Fukushima Daini nuclear power plant with its four reactors.

More reactors were in operation at Daini on March 11, 2011. A single offsite power line saved it from the catastrophe that befell Daiichi, where offsite power lines were lost to the earthquake and the emergency diesel generators were lost to the tsunami. With six reactors (three in operation) and seven spent-fuel pools at Daiichi, the four operating reactors and four pools at Daini, and one reactor and pool at the Tokai nuclear plant closer to Tokyo, then–prime minister Naoto Kan and then–chief cabinet secretary Yukio Edano admitted they had feared a "demonic chain reaction" of reactor meltdowns and pool fires. If that scenario had played out, 30 million people would have been evacuated from Tokyo—a situation akin to what filmmaker Akira Kurosawa envisioned in his 1990 film *Dreams*, where atomic reactors are seen exploding behind Mount Fuji.

The reactors at Fukushima Daiichi were General Electric Mark I boiling-water reactors, which ties the disaster to the United States. Yet our nuclear involvement in Japan stretches back seventy years to when Enrico Fermi fired up the world's first atomic reactor, the Chicago Pile-1, as part of the Manhattan Project. The original plan was to build the prototype reactor twenty miles outside downtown Chicago where the original Argonne National Laboratory was located. But there was no time, and Fermi proceeded to launch the reactor at the University of Chicago on the edge of downtown Chicago. He did not even inform the president of the university. He had convinced his superiors that it would be safe, but he took some precautions. He assigned some graduate students to a "suicide squad" tasked with pouring a chemical solution on the pile in the event of a mishap. He also stationed a man who came to be known as the Safety Control Rod Axe Man (SCRAM), who could use an axe to sever a rope holding the control rod by a pulley, causing it to fall into the out-of-control reactor. The term SCRAM has stuck in the nuclear power industry. However, as we saw at Fukushima, you can SCRAM a reactor when a 9.0 earthquake strikes, but the decay heat is enough to lead to a meltdown if you cannot cool the cores.

J. Robert Oppenheimer and General Leslie Groves tested the plutonium bomb, code-named Trinity, at Alamogordo, New Mexico, on July 16, 1945. It was the precursor of the bomb dropped on Nagasaki on August 9. They did not have to test the uranium bomb, dropped on Hiroshima on August 6, because there was no doubt that it would work. Later, the U.S. government would list the Hiroshima and Nagasaki atom bomb blasts as "tests," which, in a ghoulish sense, they were, especially since they were not needed to end the war. Such "tests" would continue.

The tests in the Pacific Ocean were part of a Cold War arms race with the Soviets. Eisenhower gave his "Atoms for Peace" speech at the United Nations on December 8, 1953, which was pure propaganda. Uranium mining, milling, processing, and enrichment were to be expanded, but the difficulty lay in how to sell it to the American people. In short, they put a smiley face on all things nuclear. This was at a time when the first "civilian" atomic reactor had not yet fired up in Shippingport, Pennsylvania, under the direction of Hyman Rickover. Most of the uranium in this country had been feeding the arms race for years, and even decades, before the commercial industry significantly entered the picture in the late 1960s and early 1970s. Then the uranium supply started to shift over to fuel those reactors.

Castle Bravo was the code name for the first of a series
of hydrogen bomb tests that the United States carried out
at locations such as the Bikini Atoll on March 1, 1954. The
Bravo test did not proceed as planned. One of the bomb's
designers, Edward Teller, and other scientists miscalculated
the yield of this explosion. They expected a five-megaton
blast. Instead, there was a fifteen-megaton blast. It is still
the worst incident of radiological contamination in the
history of U.S. nuclear weapons testing. A Japanese tuna-
fishing boat, the *Lucky Dragon #5*, was unfortunately not
very far away. It was initially outside the zone that had been
declared off-limits, but later the United States redrew the
zone. The boat was well within danger. Over time, around
half of the crew of twenty-three died of their radiation exposures. One of the deaths occurred within a matter of
months, and it led to an antinuclear groundswell in Japan,
including a petition drive with tens of millions of signatures
protesting against atomic bomb and hydrogen bomb tests.
A million signatures came from the Hiroshima area alone.
The United States was concerned. There were fears that
even the Soviet Union or Communist China could take advantage of the situation, in a bid to win the loyalty of post-
war Japan.

A part of the U.S. response to shore up the Atoms for
Peace campaign was to deploy the CIA in Japan. Lewis
Strauss, the head of the Atomic Energy Commission, and
his agency took a lead role in downplaying the signifi-

cance of the radioactive seafood contamination in Japan. Matsutaro Shoriki, a former "Class A" war criminal suspect and then media mogul known as Japan's Citizen Kane, controlled one of the largest newspapers and one of the largest television stations in Japan. He had high ambitions for political office and helped found the Liberal Democratic Party, which went on to rule Japan for half a century. In 2006, it was found that he had been working with the CIA. One of his assignments was to sell nuclear power to the Japanese people, and he did it with a passion. Among the first companies to take advantage of the situation was a company Shoriki worked for. General Dynamics had entered the nuclear business early, but General Electric was not far behind.

And so Japan's infamous "nuclear village" with its Plutonium Boy mascot was born. A complex of the nuclear power industry, electric utility companies, political leaders, government promotional and regulatory agencies, public relations firms, academics, labor unions, and local officials, it grew over time into one of the most powerful political and economic forces in Japan. Through well-funded propaganda campaigns often targeted at children, it maintained the "nuclear safety myth" until it was forever shattered by the Fukushima nuclear catastrophe.

There have been a total of about 140 commercial atomic reactors in the United States, 100 of which are still running. There are also more than twenty reactors in Canada. Atomic

Japan is third only to the United States and France with its fifty-eight reactors. (Japan had fifty-four commercial reactors, before the Fukushima Daiichi catastrophe wrecked four of them.) Japan also has a problem-plagued experimental fast-breeder reactor, Monju, named after the bodhisattva Manjusri in an attempt to win pro-nuclear favor from Fukui Prefecture's Buddhists. Fukui alone has a remarkable number of reactors—fourteen on a short stretch of coastline, the most of any prefecture in Japan. A remarkable testament to the antinuclear movement and people of Japan is that only two reactors have been restarted since the country's nuclear plants were taken offline for safety checks and upgrades, refueling, and/or maintenance repairs after the beginning of the Fukushima nuclear catastrophe, and those—at Oi, in Fukui—only for a limited time. Meanwhile, there are numerous reactors in the United States that are vulnerable to near-term, permanent shutdown. We need to shut the reactors down before they melt down.

The history of nuclear accidents in the United States and Japan demonstrates some remarkable parallels.

Worker overexposure: In 1981, three hundred workers were exposed to excessive levels of radiation after a fuel rod ruptured at the Tsuruga Nuclear Power Plant in Fukui Prefecture. This was reminiscent of an incident in the 1970s when a mixed-oxide plutonium (MOX) fuel rod broke at an experimental reactor at Big Rock Point in Michigan, releasing a large quantity of hazardous radioactivity. A similar incident occurred in 2009 at one of the largest nuclear power plants in North America—the Bruce Nuclear Generating Station on the Great Lakes in Canada. Hundreds of workers wearing no respiratory protection were exposed to alpha-particle radiation when they were grinding through contaminated pipes. There are currently nine reactors on the site, and its owner, Ontario Power Generation, is also proposing to place a "low- to intermediate-level" radioactive waste dump for all of Ontario's twenty reactors less than a mile from Lake Huron. In addition, half a dozen nearby communities, mostly populated by Bruce workers, have volunteered to host a high-level radioactive waste dump for all of Canada. These proposals endanger the Great Lakes, which contain 20 percent of the world's surface freshwater, providing drinking water to 40 million people in North America.

Sodium fires: Monju suffered a major fire in 1995. There was widespread public outrage when it emerged that the Power Reactor and Nuclear Fuel Development Corporation, the semigovernmental agency then running Monju, had tried to cover up the extent of the accident and damage. The cover-up included falsifying reports and editing videotape taken immediately after the accident, as well as issuing a gag order on employees. Fermi Unit 1 in Monroe County,

Michigan, famous for the partial meltdown of its reactor core on October 5, 1966, also suffered a sodium fire, as well as tritium leaks, in 2008. What is remarkable is that it had permanently shut down in 1972. These Fermi 1 accidents were decommissioning accidents. The meltdown was covered up for nearly a decade until the publication of John G. Fuller's book *We Almost Lost Detroit.*

Reprocessing facility accidents: On March 11, 1997, forty workers were exposed to radiation at a Tokaimura reprocessing facility in Japan. In the United States, a commercial and military reprocessing facility that operated from 1966 to 1972 at West Valley in Buffalo, New York, experienced so many incidents of fire, leaking, and worker overexposure that it only managed one year's worth of reprocessing. The cost of cleaning the site up is between 10 and 27 billion dollars. If it is not cleaned up, it will erode into Lakes Erie and Ontario.

Inadvertent criticalities: Fermi Unit 2, which is the largest GE Mark I boiling-water reactor in the world—the same design as at Fukushima Daiichi, only nearly as large as Units 1 and 2 put together—experienced an inadvertent criticality in 1985. Michael Keegan at Don't Waste Michigan uncovered the accident and the reactor was shut down for three years because it did not yet have a permit to operate. Luckily no one was hurt.

On June 18, 1999, during an inspection, operators were to perform an emergency control rod insertion on Shika

Unit 1 in Japan's Ishikawa Prefecture. Due to improper procedure, instead of inserting one rod into the reactor, three rods were withdrawn. For the next fifteen minutes, the reactor was in a dangerous criticality state. This event was covered up and not revealed until March 15, 2007. A second, much more serious Tokaimura nuclear accident— a fatal inadvertent criticality—occurred on September 30, 1999, as three workers were preparing a small batch of fuel for an experimental fast-breeder reactor. It resulted in two workers' deaths, and the exposure of hundreds of other workers and local residents to radioactivity doses above so-called permissible levels.

Cover-ups: In 2000, three TEPCO executives were forced to resign after the revelation that in 1989 the company had ordered an employee to edit out video footage showing cracks in nuclear plant steam pipes. In August 2002, a widespread falsification scandal led to the temporary shutdown of all of TEPCO's seventeen atomic reactors: company officials had falsified inspection records and attempted to hide cracks in reactor vessel shrouds in thirteen reactors. Nevertheless, TEPCO was allowed to restart the reactors. According to Aileen Mioko Smith at the Japanese organization Green Action, there was another cover-up in Japan that was brought to light by the Japanese antinuclear movement: in 1999, British Nuclear Fuels' MOX fuel arrived in Japan with falsified quality assurance documentation, which caused a major delay in plutonium fuel loading in Japan. Unfortunately, the first MOX was loaded into Fukushima Daiichi Unit 3 just six months prior to the March 11 catastrophe. Unit 3 suffered the biggest explosion of all.

Another cover-up, in the United States, took place at Davis-Besse, Ohio, which had a massive corrosion hole in the lid of its reactor in 2002 and came within three-sixteenths of an inch of breaching the seven-inch carbon steel lid. Video footage was edited before the NRC saw it, but the commission had photographic evidence of a lava-like stream of boric acid crystals and rust coming off the lid. Despite this, no regulatory action was taken. The finger-prints of former NRC chairman Richard Meserve were all over this near-disaster. Junior inspectors at the NRC wanted to shut the plant down for inspections. Instead, Meserve and others in senior management at NRC allowed the reactor to continue operating. The office of the inspector general later reported that NRC had prioritized company profits over public safety. Meserve resigned shortly afterward yet is still called upon to present on nuclear safety matters, even in Tokyo. He has served on numerous legal and scientific communities over the years, including many established by the National Academies of Sciences (NAS) and Engineering (NAE). Tipped off about Meserve's membership on two for-profit nuclear utility corporate boards—at Pacific Gas & Electric, which owns Diablo Canyon nuclear power plant in California, and Luminant, which owns Comanche Peak in Texas—Beyond Nuclear successfully demanded Meserve's recusal from the board's analysis of cancer risks in populations near nuclear facilities.

Steam explosions: At Mihama 3 in Fukui Prefecture, four workers were killed by a steam explosion on the 2004 anniversary of the dropping of the bomb on Nagasaki. The subsequent investigation revealed a significant lack of systematic inspections at Japanese nuclear power plants.

Surry Nuclear Power Plant in Virginia has experienced two separate accidents, in 1972 and 1986. The former killed two workers, the latter four—the single largest immediate loss of human life at a U.S. nuclear power plant. Surry is also infamous for experimenting with various types of dry cask storage. There have been leaks of inert heat transfer gas out of one seal and possibly out of a second. Complete seal failure leakage would allow oxygen to enter the cask and the waste to overheat, leading to corrosion or deterioration of the irradiated nuclear fuel inside.

Nonfatal radioactive steam releases: In 2006, Fukushima Daiichi itself experienced a radioactive steam release. An especially controversial incident was in January 2012, when radioactive steam was released from a failed steam-generating tube at San Onofre in Southern California. As a result, the two units in San Onofre were shut down. Extensive, dangerous tube degradation was discovered in nearly new replacement steam generators, which had cost $671 million. This was due to faulty design and fabrication performed by Mitsubishi Heavy Industries of Japan. In June 2013, Southern California

Edison announced the permanent shutdown of both reactors. The total cost of the fiasco is now in the billions of dollars, with legal disputes as to who will pay.

Earthquakes: On July 16, 2007, a severe earthquake measuring 6.8 on the Richter scale hit the region where TEPCO's Kashiwazaki-Kariwa nuclear power plant is located. Radioactive water spilled into the Sea of Japan, a transformer caught on fire, and radioactive waste containers were jostled and overturned. The plant, with seven reactors, is the single largest in the world. Although a small number of Kashiwazaki-Kariwa's reactors had returned to service by March 11, 2011, the entire plant was shut down shortly thereafter, and it remains shut down to the present day. This is a testament to popular resistance on the local level and the hard work of a burgeoning antinuclear movement, including unprecedentedly frequent and large-scale protests, including some numbering hundreds of thousands. Prime Minister Abe remains determined to restart reactors, despite the risks.

Entergy's Indian Point nuclear plant, in Buchanan, New York, is located immediately adjacent to fault lines that were discovered long after it was constructed. Seismologists at Columbia University confirmed their existence in 2008. The NRC was then forced to admit that this is probably the most vulnerable nuclear power plant in the United States to earthquakes, which it was not constructed to withstand. The Diablo Canyon atomic reactors in California are also vulnerable to earthquakes but are more sturdily built because engineers knew of the proximity of the San Andreas Fault. But in recent years, previously unknown fault lines immediately adjacent to Diablo Canyon have also been discovered.

Reactor pressure vessel embrittlement: Another risk, faced specifically by pressurized water reactors, is reactor pressure vessel embrittlement due to the neutron bombardment of the approximately eight-inch thickness of a reactor pressure vessel over years and decades. The impurities in the metal can create cracks that can line up, decreasing the metal's ductility. If the emergency core cooling systems are ever activated, as the final line of defense to prevent a meltdown, the thermal shock of the temperature decrease, combined with the very high pressure, can fracture these vessels, like a hot glass under cold water. If that happens, there will be an irreparable loss of core coolant. There would be no contingency in place to prevent a core meltdown. Genkai 1 in Saga Prefecture on Kyushu, and Entergy's Palisades in Michigan, have the worst embrittled RPVs in Japan and the United States, respectively.

Radioactive waste leaks: The single largest risk of radioactive waste leaks at the present time is at Fukushima Daiichi Unit 4. The reactor building is severely damaged from the March 2011 hydrogen explosion and is at risk of collapse. If this were to happen, the many hundreds of irradiated nuclear fuel assemblies in the storage pool could erupt into a radioactive inferno. The radioactive releases would dwarf what has already escaped into the environment. It is worth noting, however, that U.S. high-level radioactive waste storage pools contain many times the amount of radioactive waste as at Fukushima Daiichi Unit 4, and a high-level radioactive waste fire in the United States could unleash a catastrophe because just as in Japan the storage pools are not located within robust radiological containment structures.

There have been high-level radioactive waste leaks in the United States, too. The U.S. Department of Energy has revealed that six underground storage tanks containing high-level radioactive waste liquids and sludge are leaking up to 1,000 gallons per year close to the Columbia River bordering Washington and Oregon. The waste comes from military reprocessing and the U.S. Cold War nuclear arsenal. Hanford has a total of 177 tanks, containing 53 million gallons of liquid high-level radioactive waste. Of the 177, 149 are single shelled, meaning the waste is leaking directly into the environment. The remaining tanks are double shelled, yet these too have also started to leak. The Hanford site's high-level radioactive waste must be transferred to new, state-of-the-art double-shelled tanks. Vitrification (solidification into glass logs) of the liquids and sludge must be carried out as a priority in order to stabilize the high-level radioactive waste for the longer term.

On the commercial side, the list of confirmed leaks of tritium and other hazardous radionuclides from high-level radioactive waste has grown at an alarming rate. The following storage pools have been documented to have leaked into soil, groundwater, and surface waters: Hatch, Georgia; Indian Point, New York; Palo Verde, Arizona; Salem, New Jersey; Brookhaven National Lab's High Flux Beam Reactor, New York; BWX Technologies, Virginia; San Onofre, California; Seabrook, New Hampshire; and Watts Bar, Tennessee.

The NRC admits to additional leaks from high-level radioactive waste storage pools in the United States, but claims "leaked spent fuel pool water was contained within spent fuel pool leakage-collection systems." These were at Crystal River, Florida; Davis-Besse, Ohio; Diablo Canyon, California; Duane Arnold, Iowa; and Hope Creek, New Jersey. Leaks were reported at Kewaunee, Wisconsin, but the NRC notes only "white boric acid deposits, possible boric acid, observed on the wall and ceiling of the waste drumming room adjacent to the spent fuel pool."

Additional leaks into soil, groundwater, and surface waters have been reported at most operating reactors, according to Beyond Nuclear's Paul Gunter in his 2010 report "Leak First, Fix Later." Beyond Nuclear's "Routine Radioactive Releases from U.S. Nuclear Power Plants" report shows how radioactivity emissions into air and water are a "permitted," "regular" occurrence at every stage of the uranium fuel chain, including at atomic reactors. "Permissible" or "allowable" should not be confused with "safe," as every exposure to radioactivity, no matter how low the dose, increases a person's risk of developing cancer, and such risks accumulate over a lifetime. The NAS has confirmed this in multiple reports over decades.

False solutions to the radioactive waste dilemma abound. The only real solution to the problem of radioactive waste is to stop producing it in the first place. The block in Japan on restarting all reactors—other than the reactor at Oi in Fukui Prefecture—has meant that no radioactive waste has been generated there for some time now. In the United States, the permanent shutdowns at Kewaunee, Wisconsin; Crystal River, Florida; and San Onofre 2 and 3 in California, and the announced closure of Vermont Yankee by the end of 2014, mean that high-level radioactive waste will no longer be generated at any of these sites. These are the first reactor shutdowns in the United States in fifteen years and are a testament to the tireless activism of the antinuclear movement.

For the high-level radioactive waste that already exists, U.S. environmental groups have long called for hardened on-site storage (HOSS) as an interim measure to empty dangerous storage pools and to upgrade dry cask storage in order to fortify radioactive waste against possible attack and prevent its leakage for the long term. HOSS also aims to prevent unnecessary centralized interim storage risks, including reprocessing.

Meanwhile, the U.S. nuclear power industry is seeking to offload responsibility for high-level radioactive waste onto the American taxpayer. U.S. senators, such as Ron Wyden

(D-OR), Dianne Feinstein (D-CA), Lamar Alexander (R-TN), Lisa Murkowski (R-AK), and Angus King (I-ME)—as well as the Department of Energy and its Blue Ribbon Commission on America's Nuclear Future—are proposing "consolidated interim storage" by 2021, which would create an unprecedented number of risks in the form of trucks, trains, and barges carrying irradiated nuclear fuel through many states.

Under the Yucca Mountain dump plan, which the Obama administration has wisely canceled, the Department of Energy proposed barging 111 containers of high-level radioactive waste from the atomic reactor at Oyster Creek up the Jersey shore, past Staten Island, to Newark. Fifty-eight barges were to carry high-level radioactive waste down the Hudson River from Indian Point to Jersey City, passing close to Manhattan. Forty-two barges were to carry high-level radioactive waste from Connecticut through the Long Island Sound to New Haven.

The Savannah River Site in South Carolina and the Waste Isolation Pilot Plant in New Mexico—already burdened by military radioactive waste contamination and dumping—are high on the list of proposed commercial irradiated nuclear fuel dumps. So too are Native American reservations, a blatant example of radioactive racism. The Dresden nuclear power plant, southwest of Chicago in Morris, Illinois, might also be a candidate as it already stores nearly three thousand tons of irradiated nuclear fuel at its three reactors and is immediately adjacent to General Electric–Hitachi Morris's storage pool—a reprocessing facility that due to a major design flaw never operated.

If irradiated nuclear fuel is consolidated at the Savannah River Site, it would be that much easier to reprocess. So far, a broad and diverse coalition in the United States has fended off major efforts to revive reprocessing, citing nuclear weapons proliferation risks, environmental risks, and its exorbitant costs. Japanese researchers and activists, such as Masa Takubo and Dr. Tadahiro Katsuta, have also sought alternatives to reprocessing, such as employing dry cask storage.

The United States and Japan have Mark I and II reactors in common. Both are catastrophically flawed General Electric boiling-water reactor designs. As a cost-saving measure, the radiological containments are too small and too weak, as was plainly apparent at Fukushima Daiichi. Numerous people have long warned of its defects, including AEC safety officer Stephen Hanauer in 1972; the "GE Three" whistleblowers Gregory C. Minor, Richard B. Hubbard, and Dale G. Bridenbaugh in 1976; and Harold Denton, a top safety official at NRC, in 1986. Yet there are still twenty-three Mark I reactors operating in the United States, and eight similarly designed Mark II reactors. These must be shut down before they melt down, especially given the collusion in Japan between the government and the power industry, which was identified by the Japanese diet's independent investigation as the root cause of the Fukushima disaster. A very similar collusion exists in the United States between the nuclear power industry, the NRC, and elected officials. Gene Stilp, a Harrisburg, Pennsylvania, resident and long-time nuclear watchdog, took part in an antinuclear protest in Michigan in 1999 with a banner that read, THREE MILE ISLAND, CHORNOBYL, WHERE NEXT? Of course, the answer to that was Fukushima.

15

Post-Fukushima Food Monitoring

Cindy Folkers

Radiation from Fukushima reached the United States directly, including the radioactive isotopes iodine-131, cesium-134, and cesium-137. Iodine-131, due to its eight-day half-life, was a health threat in the first few months after the accident began. While it no longer poses a new exposure risk, those who were exposed to iodine-131 during this early time should continue to be monitored for diseases, such as thyroid disorders, which could manifest years after this initial exposure. Cesium-134 has a half-life of about two years and cesium-137 a half-life of about thirty years. Both will continue to pose a health risk for a few decades (cesium-134) to hundreds of years (cesium-137). Going forward, we must assess how cesium becomes concentrated or biomagnified in the environment over the long term and where it might enter our food supply.

Certain types of radiation that would be less damaging outside our bodies can become much more damaging if inhaled or ingested since there is nothing inside our bodies to block this radioactivity. Each disintegration, or "hit," represented by a becquerel, may cause damage and disease. Because some radiation is blocked more easily, it is challenging to measure certain radionuclides inside food if this is the only type of radiation that they emit.

In general, gamma radiation is easier to measure because it travels more easily through most material, including the flesh of an apple or a fish. This makes gamma radiation the obvious choice for testing because the food samples require less preparation.

The radionuclide cesium-137 emits a gamma ray and is therefore the radionuclide most often measured. Even if you do not detect the cesium gamma, this does not mean that the food does not contain other radioisotopes that are of concern, such as strontium-90 or plutonium-239. In fact, as Fukushima continues to spew radioactive isotopes, concern is growing among experts that in addition to cesium, other radioisotopes, such as strontium-90, will start to appear in greater quantities, further threatening our ocean food supply. Measuring food for just gamma radiation therefore has serious limitations, but it is a reasonable starting point in any food-testing program.

Fukushima is not the only source of cesium contamination. We have been exposed to man-made radiation for generations from a number of different sources. Atomic bomb blasts worldwide have released 954 petabecquerels of cesium, while every nuclear power reactor releases radionuclides into the water and air as part of its operating plan. It does not take an accident to release this material, although there have been plenty of those. A total release amount for cesium-137 and cesium-134 for the U.S. nuclear power reactor fleet is currently unavailable and would have to be calculated. It would be based on questionable effluent-release data collected by the nuclear power industry, not independent parties.

Chornobyl released 85 quadrillion becquerels of cesium-137 with a margin of 26 petabecquerels or 26 quadrillion becquerels. Fukushima released into the air and ocean 500 quadrillion becquerels of noble gases, according to a TEPCO press release. Meanwhile, highly contaminated water from the ruined reactors continues to be released with no sign that it will stop, and in fact, for some isotopes, such as strontium-90, the releases appear to be increasing. TEPCO has underestimated the initial releases from Fukushima, and there is no evidence that they are being truthful about current releases. These releases continue with no sign that TEPCO has control of the situation and with former nuclear officials from the United States encouraging them to release all of the contaminated water into the Pacific.

There have been a number of food-testing programs. Vital Choice and Eden are private companies that pay to have their products tested. The Berkeley Department of Nuclear Engineering ran about 115 total samples, all of which were from California and mostly from 2011. The U.S. Food and Drug Administration, the Environmental Protection Agency, and the Department of Energy have monitored food, while the National Oceanic and Atmospheric Administration keeps an eye on any contamination that might reach the *kuroshio* ocean current, which is a fast track to the California Pacific coast, and may start monitoring California coast seawater and sediment. Universities and institutes have done limited testing but need more funding to continue.

These programs have a number of shortcomings. Most samples are only tested for gamma-emitting radionuclides. Testing has been seriously curtailed now even though Fukushima is still spewing radiation and the contamination is becoming entrenched. The EPA was criticized by the inspector general because 20 percent of its radiation monitors in the United States (RadNet) were out of service when the Fukushima catastrophe began. Furthermore, sampling a piece of food every once in a while gives you no real idea of the scope of possible contamination or bioaccumulation and does not pinpoint any potential radiation hot spots.

In other words, the testing of U.S. foodstuffs is inadequate. The U.S. limit for cesium of 1,200 becquerels per kilogram is too high and is not binding, so the FDA can decide to act or not at any level of cesium contamination. It is little different from having no standard or limit at all. By comparison, Japan's limit is 100 becquerels per kilogram, meaning that food too contaminated for Japan can be imported to the United States. No one has yet explained why children in the United States are allowed to ingest twelve times more radioactive poison than children in Japan. In any case, the release of contaminated food information to the public in the United States is at best paltry, if it is released at all.

After the initial release from Fukushima, radioactive iodine levels in Californian kelp were found to be significantly
higher than before Fukushima. The researchers who conducted this study did not test the kelp for cesium, but they
should, especially since kelp provides a food source for fish
and there is concern that contamination will be concentrated
in fish that feed on it.

California grass was found to contain 14 becquerels of
cesium-134 and cesium-137 per kilogram. Grass, like kelp, is
the beginning of a potential biomagnification chain, which
could concentrate cesium in cattle. As the Berkeley monitoring site put it, "for understanding the time-dependence of
food chain results, the grass and soil is what to look at."

Pistachios that were grown in California and shipped to
a Japanese supermarket were tested. They were found to
contain 18 becquerels of cesium-134 and cesium-137 per
kilogram. Beef raised in Japan was tested and approved for
sale and then recalled, but not before it was fed to Japanese
schoolchildren. This beef had contamination levels between
650 and 2,300 becquerels of cesium per kilogram. All of this
beef could have been sold to the United States and the FDA
may not have pulled it because, even though a contamination
level of 2,300 becquerels of cesium per kilogram is above the
FDA limit, this limit is not binding, meaning the FDA can
choose to do nothing. Meanwhile, 162 kilograms of green
tea were shipped to France from Japan and rejected because
of the level of contamination, 1,038 becquerels of cesium per
kilogram. The United States would have accepted this tea.

Bluefin tuna swam all the way across the Pacific and reached the California coast retaining cesium-134 and cesium-137. Canada's cesium limit is 1,000 becquerels of cesium per kilogram and news reports expressed concern that Canada will also import highly contaminated fish from Japan—a concern that the United States should also share. Ocean life researchers were also concerned that contamination was higher in 2012 than it had been in 2011. This fits with cesium's tendency to biomagnify. We need more testing and we need to think about how to test over a longer time frame, not just a few years. Testing in Japan recently found that wild blueberry jam imported from Italy, made from blueberries grown in Bulgaria, was contaminated above Japan's 100-becquerels-per-kilogram cesium limit at approximately 140–160 becquerels per kilogram. Most likely its contamination is from the Chornobyl nuclear explosion, which points to the many sources of radioactive contamination, only one of which is Fukushima. Had a newspaper not tested the jam and publicly pressured the Japanese government to remove it from shelves, the preserves would still be available for sale. Meanwhile, this brand is sold in the United States as well and it carries the organic label. It is likely that U.S. parents who are trying to feed their children a higher-quality product, like organic preserves, are unwittingly and with no small measure of irony subjecting them to this radioactivity.

So how should we think about these contamination levels? What does the 1,200-becquerels-per-kilogram limit actually mean? Remember two things: there is no safe level of radiation, and cesium-134 and cesium-137 did not exist in nature before we created and released them.

The International Commission on Radiological Protection (ICRP) recommends how much radiation exposure can be tolerated by humans, and governments often follow these recommendations when setting standards. Nonetheless, when even very small amounts of cesium are ingested routinely, they can build up to unexpected levels in the body. After about three years, ingesting 10 becquerels of cesium-137 per day will cause a buildup of over 1,400 becquerels of cesium-137 in your body. For a child who weighs about 30 kilograms (66 pounds), this would be about 50 becquerels of cesium-137 per kilogram in the body. In studies of post-Chornobyl Belarus, cardiac abnormalities were seen in children whose bodies contained 10 to 30 becquerels of cesium per kilogram. Irreversible myocardial pathologies were observed at 50 becquerels per kilogram. Additional observed pathologies at these low levels included hormone imbalances, angina, diabetes, and hypertension.

In addition to these diseases, as cesium passes out of the body, its radioactivity damages the kidneys and bladder and the body's ability to rid itself of the cesium. This could mean the total amount of cesium in a body could rise over time from chronic ingestion.

The high U.S. limits seem to be part of an official policy to encourage people to accept an increasingly radioactive food supply. Consider this from the ICRP report "Application of the Commission's Recommendations to the Protection of

People Living in Long-Term Contaminated Areas After a Nuclear Accident or a Radiation Emergency": "There may be situations where a sustainable agriculture economy is not possible without placing contaminated food on the market. As such foods will be subject to market forces, this will necessitate an effective communication strategy to overcome the negative reactions from consumers outside the contaminated areas." Their plan consists not of informing the public about what these contamination levels are so that we can decide for ourselves what is or is not appropriate. It consists instead of convincing us that man-made radiation in small doses is not harmful.

Beyond Nuclear, in coalition with other groups that are part of the Fukushima Fallout Awareness Network (FFAN), are petitioning the FDA for a binding contamination limit of 5 becquerels of cesium-134 and/or cesium-137 per kilogram instead of the current nonbinding 1,200 becquerels per kilogram. A 5-becquerels-per-kilogram limit is also close to that recommended by the International Physicians for the Prevention of Nuclear War (IPPNW) in their report "Calculated Fatalities from Radiation: Officially Permissible Limits for Radioactively Contaminated Food in the European Union and Japan." Interestingly, each of the groups had arrived at this limit independent of the other, using two different methods of assessment. We are also asking that food testing be widespread and that the data be recorded in a publicly available database no matter what the cesium contamination level. If constructed properly, this could inform research on cesium mobility/biomagnification in the environment. It could be useful for consumers and researchers. The FDA petition process could drag on for a year or more and is, at the time of writing, still under way. In the meantime, there are a number of ongoing independent citizen monitoring attempts in the United States and Canada. At this point these are a patchwork of efforts born out of frustration at official inaction. We are attempting to coordinate a more integrated, scientifically rigorous structure, which would help ensure our food security by providing knowledge of which food is less contaminated or not contaminated at all.

In 2013, the American Medical Association called for testing seafood consumed in the United States for man-made radioactivity. Yet if the testing is based on the FDA cesium limit, we have circled back to the original problem: how is it all right to subject American children to twelve times more man-made radioactive poison than children in Japan? These limits are based on what is best for the nuclear industry. Clearly nothing else counts.

When I first started collecting information on a recommended level for cesium contamination in food, 5 becquerels per kilogram was suggested. Through my research, I concluded that this limit, although it appears low, is still reasonable because cesium concentrates and biomagnifies in the environment through natural processes. Cesium releases have exposed generations of humans, and we do not know the multigenerational damage it may already have caused. Studies in Belarus have indicated damage at very low levels in children, and the ICRP has admitted that even small amounts of cesium can bioaccumulate in our bodies to potentially damaging levels.

There is still a lack of publicly available information on cesium levels in food and we have no reliable estimate on how much has been or is being released. What little we know is worrisome. It is no longer just a question of which catastrophe or routine release is to blame for contamination. It is a question of the totality of radioactive contamination and the damage caused across generations.

16

Gender Matters in the Atomic Age

Mary Olson

Nuclear disasters have a beginning but no end. To quote Physicians for Social Responsibility, prevention is the only cure. We have to move collectively, as a society, toward prevention and precaution as the basis of policy, and for that to happen, more women must get involved.

I am a public speaker, and about four years ago I started receiving questions from women in the audience about how radiation affects women to a greater degree than men. I called one of my mentors, the late Dr. Rosalie Bertell, because despite having been in this field for eighteen years, I did not have answers. Rosalie directed me first to a report that was out of print, and then to the National Academy of Sciences report *Health Risks from Exposure to Low Levels of Ionizing Radiation: BEIR VII Phase 2* (2006). My analysis of the data in the report revealed that over a lifetime, women who were exposed to radiation suffered 40 to 60 percent more harm (measured as cancer and fatal cancer) than men who were exposed to the same dose. For every two men who get cancer, three women get cancer; men get sick, but quite a few more women get sick. As Rosalie had predicted, the report did not mention this difference.

Harm from radiation is disproportionate across the life cycle. We know that primary germ cells and the embryo are far more vulnerable. The cells of fetuses and children divide more rapidly than those of adults. Dr. Alice Stewart found that the vulnerability of elderly people also increases; their repair mechanisms may not function as well as those of younger people. Some genotypes are more likely to contract radiological cancers. To this list we must now add gender: females, both juvenile and adult, are less resistant to ionizing radiation exposure. In addition to the type, amount, and duration of exposure, it matters crucially who is exposed to the radiation.

Radiation is invisible, but you can see the harm that radiation causes; indeed, we can see radiation burns (figure 16.1) to the body. We can, with a microscope, see radiation-induced chromosomal aberrations (figure 16.2) and we can also see tissue damage from plutonium. An artist's concept shows us the damage radiation can cause to DNA, reconstructed from chemical assay.

There is no safe dose of atomic radiation. It takes only a single, infinitesimal radioactive emission hitting a single cell to cause a fatal cancer. This does not happen every time— our bodies have incredible repair mechanisms—but the loss of an embryo or fetus, or even the death of an adult, are all possible outcomes from so small an event that it cannot be measured as a "dose."

The U.S. Environmental Protection Agency (EPA) safe drinking water standards say that there is no safe dose of radiation, and the U.S. Nuclear Regulatory Commission (NRC) regulations in chapter 10, part 20 of the Code of Federal Regulations, and its ALARA (As Low As Reasonably Achievable) policy, reflect this fact. This is also the conclusion of the seven BEIR reports from the National Academy of Sciences. As Dr. Bertell once said, "There is no such thing as a radiation exposure that will not do damage. There is a hundred percent possibility that there will be damage to cells. The next question is: which damage do you care about?"

When radiation impact is considered, generalizations about radiation are based on males. The first standards were established by the medical community for doctors. Later, "health physics" was created to supervise paramilitary and military personnel sent into radiation areas in the Manhattan Project. Those standards were for young, healthy males to be sent into restricted zones that were, at that time, very rare. The radiation exposure standards were not created with the view of being applied to anyone, anytime, anywhere, and since the standards do not factor in the disproportionate impact of radiation, they lead us to drastically underestimate the harm for women. Since women make up about half the population, this means an overall underestimation of radiation harm for the general populace.

Radiation exposure standards have been generalized as radioactive industries have spread. A widely used image to illustrate the breakout of radiation exposure shows the startling fact that one-fifth of an average total radiation exposure is from man-made sources. This represents a relatively large percentage that is actually an increase in radiation exposure compared to natural levels prior to the discovery of radioactivity at the end of the nineteenth century. While the chart is often used to explain away concerns about radiation exposure from nuclear energy, one must not dismiss an overall increase in exposure to ionizing radiation over the last hundred years of 25 percent (on average) overall. If any other environmental factor such as heat or rainfall were to increase by this large amount, it too would have impacts on living organisms.

The World Health Organization was the first major agency to release information about the disproportionate harm of radiation on females. In spite of its flaws, the report, called "Health Risk Assessment from the Nuclear Accident After the 2011 Great East Japan Earthquake and Tsunami," does acknowledge that radiation has different effects on males and females. They mention that for little girls exposed below the age of five, there is a 70 percent higher risk of cancer.

No research has yet determined why gender is a factor in radiation harm. Dr. Bertell hypothesized that it may be the higher percentage of reproductive tissue in the female body, since the gonads and mammary tissues are known to be radiosensitive.

Other factors like lifestyle and occupation are less likely to be operative in the 0–5 age group, where exposure to ionizing radiation produces the largest gender-based difference in outcome.

Not all radioactivity results in radiation exposure or dose, but at the moment official estimates of harm from radioactivity assume that when radioactivity impacts living tissues it is an external dose. It is important to keep in mind that internal exposure is not analogous to external exposure. Eating, drinking, and breathing in radioactivity are very different from getting an X-ray. External beta particles penetrate only about one centimeter, whereas external alpha particles bounce off the skin. If the alpha-emitting element is inhaled or ingested, so the alpha particles are hitting tissue from inside the body, estimates indicate that internal alpha particle damage is anywhere from seven to one thousand times more damaging to cell structures than is X-ray (external) exposure. Another way of saying this is that when there is no distance from the source of the alpha or beta particle to its target, the doses to the target are very much higher. The *BEIR VII* report only looks at A-bomb survivors' exposure to external ionizing radiation. There is no consideration of contaminated areas: food, water, and air deliver cumulative, ongoing radiological exposure that is internal as well as external. We do not yet know the implications of internal versus external exposure in gender-based radiation harm. This is important because although there are a limited number of catastrophically contaminated zones like Chornobyl and Fukushima, every industrial site and mining site in the nuclear fuel chain produces wastes and contamination, impacting the local community.

Disproportionate harm from ionizing radiation to females raises many issues: medical, ethical, historical, occupational, political, legal, evolutionary, and policy or regulatory questions. All are worthy of engagement, but it is my belief that we need to protect first and study second.

17

Epidemiologic Studies of Radiation Releases from Nuclear Facilities

Steven Wing

There are two approaches to estimating the health impact of radiation releases from nuclear facilities. In risk assessment we begin by estimating the radiation doses for a population. Then we multiply the number of people at each dose level by a value that represents the estimated number of excess cases of disease that will develop over time for a population exposed to that amount of radiation. The numbers of excess cases at each dose level are summed to get a total, which is the estimated impact of radiation releases on that disease.

The other method is epidemiology, which involves monitoring the occurrence of disease in populations exposed to different levels of radiation. The amount of excess disease due to radiation is estimated by direct observation about the past rather than projection into the future based on assumptions. Epidemiology is modeled after experiments in which subjects are randomly assigned to be exposed to radiation and compared to unexposed subjects. However, human experiments on ionizing radiation are unethical, therefore radiation epidemiology has focused on disease rates among patients exposed to medical radiation, nuclear workers, people living in areas with different levels of environmental radiation, and people exposed to radiation from nuclear weapons.

The World Health Organization recently released a risk assessment for the Fukushima radiation releases that began in March 2011. Their estimates are based on population dose estimates provided in an earlier report and risks of cancer at those radiation levels derived from the Life Span Study (LSS) of survivors of the atomic bombs dropped on Hiroshima and Nagasaki. The dose assessment is incomplete as there are a number of components that the report ignores. For example, the committee chose not to assess the doses within twenty kilometers of the nuclear plant, occupational radiation exposure, doses from beta radiation emitted by gaseous releases, and in utero doses.

Radiation risk assessments are largely based on the Life Span Study (LSS) of survivors of the U.S. nuclear attacks on Hiroshima and Nagasaki. Follow-up of LSS participants did not begin until five or more years after the bombing, and many people did not survive long enough to be included. This introduced several sources of potential bias into radiation risk estimates. If mortality from the immediate effects of the bombings was related to longer-term risks, then the most radiosensitive people died before the study began, meaning that the LSS selected for healthier people with lower radiation risks than the people who were excluded. Furthermore, the LSS's monitoring of cancer incidence (new diagnoses of cancer rather than death) did not begin until 1958. Therefore, all cancers that occurred within thirteen years of exposure are omitted from LSS cancer incidence risk estimates. These caveats are routinely omitted when risk estimates from the LSS are applied to other populations.

The LSS has focused on the penetrating gamma and neutron radiation from the nuclear detonations, prompt radiation that was gone in seconds. However, fallout led people to be exposed to radioactive particles. Because the primary sites of fallout were not at ground zero, people most affected by fallout, also known as "black rain," were exposed to lower doses from prompt radiation. This would tend to raise disease rates among the LSS survivors with the lowest prompt radiation doses and create a downward bias in LSS radiation risk estimates. Despite the signing of a treaty banning atmospheric nuclear weapons testing in 1963, in large part due to concerns about health effects of fallout at great distances from aboveground tests, the impacts of fallout in the LSS have not been factored into radiation risk estimates.

A Radiation Effects Research Foundation (RERF) report on black rain was published in December 2012. The report summarizes analyses of survey responses of survivors who were asked about their exposures to fallout. Out of the 86,671 survivors in the primary analyses, approximately 12,000 said they had been exposed to black rain. For over 21,000, however, there is no information on exposure to black rain. This missing data is a major gap in the Life Span Study that has been ignored for half a century.

RERF reported on the mortality rates in the LSS between 1950 and 2003, and between 1962 and 2003, comparing people who said they had been exposed to black rain, those who said they had not, and those for whom exposure was not determined. The groups reporting exposure to black rain and no exposure to black rain had similar mortality in both time periods, but Hiroshima survivors for whom black rain exposure was unknown experienced 27 percent higher mortality, and Nagasaki survivors for whom black rain exposure was unknown experienced 46 percent higher mortality between 1950 and 2003. Excess mortality of people whose exposure to black rain was unknown occurred primarily during the period between 1950 and 1962.

In addition to fallout, another type of residual radiation that exposed the A-bomb survivors came from neutron activation near ground zero. This caused elevated levels of gamma radiation during the early hours and days after the detonations. People closest to ground zero, especially those with little shielding, did not survive to be included in the LSS, and residual radiation exposures from neutron activation was not important for them. However, many people who were farther from the hypocenter at the time of the bombings and who were not badly injured by heat, blast, and radiation moved through areas near ground zero shortly after the detonations, some of them looking for their relatives. As with black rain, to the extent that survivors with lower prompt gamma and neutron doses had more exposure to residual radiation than those with higher doses, there is a downward bias in LSS risk estimates.

All survivors were entered into follow-up on October 1, 1950, even though not all survivors completed sufficient interviews to be assigned a dose until 1965. This creates a phenomenon that epidemiologists call "immortal person time," which inflates the denominator of the disease rates for the proximal survivors, resulting in an underestimate of their disease rates and an underestimate of radiation risks. More important, survivors within three kilometers of ground zero who had insufficient information about location and shielding for calculating their radiation doses were excluded from analyses that produce radiation risk estimates, whereas none of the survivors who were more than three kilometers from ground zero were excluded because of the lack of such information. The excluded survivors had higher mortality from cancer and leukemia, especially during early years of follow-up, compared to survivors who were included. Because exclusions were made only for proximal survivors and not for distal survivors whose doses were lower, there is a downward bias in LSS radiation risk estimates. Existing statistical techniques for reducing bias from dose-related exclusions have not been used to correct LSS risk estimates.

The LSS is restricted to survivors exposed postnatally. A separate study has been conducted of A-bomb survivors exposed in utero, however due to their small numbers, this study has not been of much use for developing dose–response relationships for risk assessment. Perhaps in part for this reason, the Fukushima risk estimates of the World Health Organization did not include disease that would result from in utero exposure. However, ever since the 1950s, when Alice Stewart first showed that obstetric X-rays cause childhood cancer, it has been well known that the embryo and fetus are especially sensitive to low-dose radiation. Although the prenatal population exposed to Fukushima Daiichi emissions during the early time period following the meltdowns was small compared to those exposed postnatally, they are especially sensitive and should be included in risk assessments.

As I noted at the outset, risk assessment uses figures drawn from studies such as the LSS and dose estimates for populations to estimate radiation casualties in populations whose disease incidence has not been quantified. Biases in radiation effects such as those in the LSS affect risk estimation. In contrast, epidemiologic studies such as the LSS directly estimate relationships between radiation and disease; however, they can only evaluate effects after they have occurred.

I started working on radiation epidemiology in 1988 when I was assigned to lead a study of the mortality of workers employed at one of the first nuclear weapons plants, the Oak Ridge National Laboratory in eastern Tennessee. The workers' radiation doses had been monitored from very early on with individual dosimeters. I was told that we would not find any radiation effects in this population because the doses were too low, so my first clash with the dominant wisdom in this field was when we did see dose–response relationships: the higher the readings on the badges, the higher the cancer death rates of the workers. I had been told this was impossible, and yet there it was.

The disaster at Chornobyl was followed by similarly dismissive rhetoric regarding risk estimates. In a 1991 document, five years after the explosion of the Chornobyl reactor, the International Atomic Energy Agency stated: "On the basis of the doses estimated by the project teams and currently accepted radiation risk estimates, future increases over the natural incidence of cancers or hereditary effects would be difficult to discern even with large and well-designed long term epidemiological studies." Since that time a large number of epidemiologic studies have documented increases in cancer from Chornobyl's radiation releases. As in the Oak Ridge study, this prediction was made based on a risk assessment that used assumptions from the LSS.

Another nuclear event where we were told that there were no cancer effects possible was the partial meltdown of the Three Mile Island Unit 2 reactor in 1979. Many people who lived close to the plant reported symptoms such as reddening of the skin, nausea, vomiting, and hair loss, as well as the deaths of pets and animals. Those people were told that their symptoms were due to stress.

I started working on this issue because of a lawsuit that involved several thousand people. I first looked into stress, but my assessment of the medical literature was that the reports did not fit the scenario of stress-induced acute effects, sometimes called "mass psychogenic illness." We conducted a reanalysis of data from a prior study of cancer patients seen at area hospitals during the period 1975 to 1985 and found that the incidence of lung cancer and leukemia rose in the pathways of plumes of radioactive gases released during the meltdown. The study was designed to avoid detection bias, which is a major concern when studying a well-publicized event because people report disease earlier and receive more diagnostic tests due to publicity. Everyone in this study was within ten miles of the accident, however, and they were all exposed to the same detection bias.

Official estimates of the health impacts of routine releases of radiation from nuclear power plants project that no cancers will be observed among people who live near operating reactors. However, several studies conducted in Europe have found excess childhood cancer, and particularly leukemia among children aged 0–4, near power reactors. The largest, a German case-control study, showed that leukemia incidence more than doubled within five kilometers of power plants. The authors, however, concluded that "radiation exposure near German nuclear power plants is a factor of 1,000 to 100,000 less than annual average exposure from medical exams, therefore the observed positive distance trend remains unexplained."

These examples show how epidemiologic studies can produce evidence of radiation impacts that is not anticipated from risk assessments. There are three possible reasons for this. One possibility is that the epidemiologic studies are biased.

However, the biases in environmental and occupational epidemiology, most prominently poor exposure measurement, migration, and, in occupational studies, healthy worker effects, tend to cause under- rather than overestimation of radiation effects. A second reason why risk assessments may not agree with epidemiologic studies is that they use radiation risk estimates, such as those from the LSS, that are too low. A third reason is that there are seldom any direct measurements of human doses, especially for environmental radiation, and risk assessments will produce underestimates of disease if people are exposed to more radiation than assumed.

Energy generation is highly profitable, and nuclear power is tied to governments and corporations that created the nuclear weapons and power industries in the first place. This creates financial conflicts of interest in studies of radiation and health, especially when evidence of health effects could increase pressures to reduce radiation exposures to workers and the public, and when there could be lawsuits from exposed people who seek compensation. For example, government documents reviewed in the 1990s by the U.S. president's Advisory Committee on Human Radiation Experimentation clearly showed that fear of lawsuits and public opposition to the nuclear weapons program were important considerations in the deliberations of the Atomic Energy Commission's Advisory Committee on Biology and Medicine. Because our science is affected by our political system, we need public education, not only about radiation, but about science and about civic life.

In Fukushima, there will be extra challenges to epidemiological studies. Some of those challenges involve the fact that the earthquake and tsunami that triggered the meltdowns severely disrupted living conditions. People were relocating, their diets were affected, medical services were affected, and many thousands died. Estimating doses for individuals, which is critical in epidemiological studies and always difficult where people are not monitored for radiation exposure, is even more uncertain in the situation of such a disaster.

Radiation-exposed populations and the general public should know that research is imperfect. The scientific community must also understand that the main threat to research is a lack of critical thinking, which includes self-critical thinking. We must question authority, and especially studies that, like the LSS, are applied every day to legal and public health situations. However, it is equally important not to confuse narrowly constructed research hypotheses about the health effects of particular exposures with sweeping analyses of systemic issues of great interest, such as whether nuclear power is good public policy. Even if nuclear power is bad policy, that does not mean every study will find that radiation is associated with disease.

Public health activists promote policies based on broad principles such as peace, human rights, ecological sustainability, and social justice that promote health and prevent disease through diverse physical, biological, and social mechanisms. Although rooted in theory and evidence from many scientific disciplines, such principles are not hypotheses subject to refutation by specific studies; rather they are evolving world-views that integrate science, morality, and politics. Because of their global orientation, public health advocates may ignore or reject studies that do not appear to support their movement's goals, such as research that fails to demonstrate disease excesses among people exposed to radiation. Likewise, advocates may uncritically accept research that finds disease to be associated with radiation. This double standard undermines both science and public health by overemphasizing the importance of narrow research questions and by neglecting weaknesses of specific health studies. Because exposure assessments and epidemiologic studies can be easily designed to be insensitive to effects under investigation, they are most politically useful to industries and governments that are responsible for exposing workers and the general public. Therefore overemphasizing this type of research is not in the public interest. By discriminating between the results of narrow studies and broad policy goals, activists can better advance both science and public health.

18

Cancer Risk from Exposure to Low Levels of Ionizing Radiation

Herbert Abrams

The BEIR committee of the National Research Council published a report in 2006 that represented the latest in a series begun in 1972. Its aim was to convey the level of risk of low-level ionizing radiation. The report was widely accepted as a primary source of data for radiation risk estimates.

BACKGROUND

From the beginning of the twentieth century, not long after the discovery of radium and X-rays, it has been apparent that radiation has dual uses: it can cure cancer, and it can cause cancer. The harmful effects of large and medium doses have been amply demonstrated, but the effects of low-level ionizing radiation have been a subject of considerable controversy.

The Radiation Effects Research Foundation (RERF), formerly named the Atomic Bomb Casualty Commission, was founded in Hiroshima in 1947 in the wake of the atomic bombings of Hiroshima and Nagasaki. Its purpose is to document and understand the long-term effects of radiation exposure, and to that end, it employs about four hundred scientists working on many projects related to radiation. Its support comes from both the Japanese and the U.S. governments.

The foundation's Life Span Study, following 120,000 survivors in Hiroshima and Nagasaki, and its more detailed Adult Health Study, following 20,000 survivors, have continued for sixty-seven years. These projects are unique epidemiologic achievements, and they provide powerful evidence for evaluating cancer risk from radiation. The survivors in the Life Span Study are widely distributed by age. In 1995, 44,000 were still alive, and it is estimated that by 2020, 14,000 will be alive. All of them were under the age of twenty when they were exposed.

Beyond the RERF longitudinal database, there have been large numbers of research projects on subcellular elements, cells, animals, and humans addressing the biological effects of radiation and the mechanism of its effects.

COMPOSITION OF THE *BEIR VII* COMMITTEE OF THE NATIONAL RESEARCH COUNCIL

The sixteen-member advisory committee, of which I was a member, was appointed in 1999, and it worked together over a period of six years. The experts on the committee were drawn from five different countries and from different disciplines: epidemiology, genetics, radiology, physics, cancer biology, radiation biology, biostatistics, science, and risk communication.

PROCESS

There were many witnesses from interested and informed groups. As universities and governmental organizations (such as the EPA, NRC, and DOE), industry groups, NGOs, and activists took center stage, the atmosphere in the hearings sometimes became confrontational. Passions ran high because the stakes were high. If the report affected policy, larger risk estimates and lower permissible doses might follow. With lower estimates, there might be a relaxation of protection standards. Extensive reviews of the available literature were undertaken, and conflicting data were reconciled to the extent possible.

WHAT IS "LOW-LEVEL" IONIZING RADIATION?

The issue is complicated by many differing definitions. I have noted nineteen different estimates—all of them in refereed journals and with "low-level radiation" in the title—that encompass a range from 3,000 millisieverts down to 20 millisieverts. The committee came up with its own definition: a range from near zero to 100 millisieverts.

The committee's accepted definition of 100 millisieverts or less is about thirty to forty times the annual background radiation of 3 millisieverts that all of us are exposed to, ten times the level of a CAT scan, and a thousand times that of a chest X-ray. Approximately 65 percent of atomic bomb survivors received a low dose by our definition.

WHERE DOES THE RADIATION COME FROM?

Most of the radiation that we are exposed to comes from our natural background. Building materials, air, food, outer space, and Earth are major sources—especially of radon gas—and comprise 82 percent of human exposure. Roughly 18 percent is man-made, derived from medical X-rays (58 percent), nuclear medicine (21 percent), and consumer products, such as tobacco (16 percent). Two percent comes from nuclear fallout and 1 percent from the nuclear fuel cycle.

Over 300 million medical X-rays and over 120 million dental X-rays are performed every year. Together with CAT scans, which have contributed to higher-dose diagnostic examinations, the average annual effective dose is 0.5 millisieverts. Some exposures are higher, such as X-rays of the lower gastrointestinal tract, angiography, or interventional radiology. These range up to a level of 8 millisieverts.

The concern with CAT scans is their sequential use, especially in young people, because doses are cumulative. When performed repetitively over a number of years, they can increase the risk of cancer mortality. Radio-isotope exams are also common sources of relatively high doses.

WHAT WAS LEARNED FROM *BEIR VII*?

While the report covers many areas, the data support the presence of an increased risk of developing radiation cancer with increased exposure at low levels. The risk estimates are generally consistent with those documented in *BEIR V.*

Radiation damages DNA, causing single- and double-strand breaks and oxidative changes in the nucleotide bases. The DNA deletions and the gene and chromosome damage may be involved in the initiation of the neoplastic process. There is no evidence of a threshold below which no cellular damage occurs.

Significant excess relative risks have been determined for twelve cancers, including lung, liver, breast, prostate, stomach, colon, and thyroid cancer, as well as leukemia. The excess risk of breast cancer is almost 100 percent but for others it is above the 50 percent level.

The number of excess cases of cancer per 100,000 individuals exposed to 100 millisieverts at the age of 30 who have attained the age of 60 was estimated to be 800 in males and 1,300 in females. This is a relatively small but significant number compared with the natural incidence of solid tumors in an unexposed population.

Since this report, the results of a number of important epidemiological studies have been published. Among the 446,000 nuclear workers studied in fifteen countries in 2006, there was evidence of a 1 to 2 percent increase in levels of cancer deaths. The Techa River study is an example of the effects of a contaminated body of water, full of the waste from the Mayak nuclear weapons production center, which caused a 3 percent increase in cancer risk. A British study of 175,000 nuclear workers found that protracted radiation exposure caused higher risk. A post-2002 combination of twelve epidemiologic studies also confirmed *BEIR VII*'s conclusions.

There are countervailing approaches, such as hormesis, which suggest a beneficial effect at low doses. Interest in "the bystander effect," adaptive response, and genomic instability has been intense. The data from high-background areas in India and China have been considered by some as neutralizing the support for low-level radiation effects. All these considerations were reviewed and analyzed by the committee but were not convincing.

The one opinion that everyone shares is that we are dealing with uncertainties in this area.

Gender differences in the effects of radiation exposure were apparent, with radiation-related cancer mortality risks for women 37.5 percent higher than for men in the solid tumors. Exposure in infants, as compared to adults, was associated with three to four times the cancer risk, and female infants had almost double the risk of males. It should be noted that all of these excess relative risk figures are estimates, with a 95 percent confidence level.

Although low doses increase risk, the increase is not huge. As lifetime exposure accumulates, so does the risk. Exposure to low-level radiation at a younger age will probably initiate one excess cancer for every hundred individuals in a lifetime.

Extracting an exact signal from the noise has been one of the great problems with radiation epidemiology. High levels of radiation exposure increase the risk of heart disease, but we cannot detect any impact of low-level exposure. There was no conclusive evidence of genetic effects in the offspring of A-bomb survivors, in contrast to animal studies, which showed that increased cellular mutations in animals can be passed on to their offspring.

The *BEIR VII* advisory committee was a balanced and thoughtful group. We could draw on extensive expertise in many different fields. There was controversy, but the discussion continued and the material provided by the witnesses aided in developing a consensus. We will never have all the answers, but continued research will advance our understanding and improve the precision of our estimates.

19

The Rise and Fall of Nuclear Power

David Freeman

The atomic age started with the dropping of a bomb.

Perhaps only those alive at the time would appreciate the guilt this caused America. No one wanted to talk about whether America should or should not have dropped the bomb. But President Harry S. Truman believed we could make a blessing out of this terrible event, and Americans were deluged with the most vivid descriptions of how this awesome, godlike power would be turned to the benefit of humankind.

It's useful to examine some of the words that were said. Robert Maynard Hutchins, the president of the University of Chicago, where much of the research for the Manhattan Project was done, said that atomic power would make "heat so plentiful that it will even be used to melt snow as it falls. A very few individuals working a few hours a day at very easy tasks in the central atomic power plant will provide all the heat, light, and power required by the community and these utilities will be so cheap that their cost can hardly be reckoned." There was talk of only having to fill gas tanks once a year with a pill-sized pellet of atomic energy rather than twice a week with gas. The day would be gone when nations would fight for oil; the era of atomic energy would usher in an age of plenty.

And people believed it. It was a euphoric time.

Meanwhile, U.S. Atomic Energy Commission (AEC) chairman David Lilienthal reported to Truman, at about the time the Russians tested their bomb, that America had no stockpile of bombs. According to Lilienthal's journals, there was never any discussion of civilian nuclear power. It was an arms race. All the talk about a nuclear idyll was just talk, and in its stead came the hydrogen bomb. After all, the scientists in their secure university positions did not have to dirty their hands with pipes and pumps and the machinery of developing nuclear reactors for civilian use.

It took Hyman G. Rickover, a four-star admiral of the U.S. Navy working with a private company, to develop the Nautilus submarine—the first civilian application of nuclear power. The costs were so astronomical that it ultimately had little civilian application, but it did give people a basis for thinking that perhaps all these dreams about nuclear power had some validity to them. The period of nuclear euphoria lasted into the 1950s. The research did not produce anything. The AEC knew that they were nowhere near building a civilian reactor but they continued to make grandiose promises in order to secure funding from Congress to continue their weapons program.

The beginning of the civilian nuclear power program came in 1957, when Congress passed the Price Anderson Act. Early research on reactors proved unsuccessful, but the big breakthrough came in 1963 when General Electric made a bid to build a nuclear power plant at Oyster Creek in New Jersey. They offered a price cheaper than coal, and the AEC hailed this as the first step in the commercialization of nuclear power. It was, however, a loss-leader bid. GE had no idea what a nuclear power plant would cost. All that it knew was that it was time to start selling them. It had a turnkey deal at a price that made it competitive but that was far below the actual cost. This ushered in the era of the cost overrun. These plants were built and sold at a price that looked like it was competitive with coal, even though there has never been a nuclear power plant built that was cost-competitive in this country or anywhere else. All of a sudden, what looked like a dormant option—the cause of much lip service—was the rage.

I remember when GE came to my law firm in the 1960s and asked us to help them create a public power agency in New Jersey because they wanted to build half a dozen nuclear reactors there. Fortunately, GE's lawyers said they would be violating antitrust laws and put a stop to the plan, but that was the prevailing mind-set at the time. A year later, Peabody Coal Company came to us and said they were so afraid of nuclear power taking over the future that they did not think that coal resources in the West would be developed. They wanted to create public power agencies with low-interest money to lower the price of coal so that they might have a chance at competing.

It got worse. By the time I took over the Tennessee Valley Authority in 1976, TVA had stopped maintenance of its coal plants for years. They were going nuclear. With an armada of twelve nuclear reactors, they were writing off their coal plants. We put a billion dollars into installing scrubbers and pollution-control equipment on those plants.

AEC chairman Glenn T. Seaborg said he was certain that nuclear power was the future. He traveled to sixty nations to sell the idea of the peaceful atom as outlined in Eisenhower's famous "Atoms for Peace" speech to the United Nations on December 8, 1953. Most people believed him. The first time I went to Israel, I asked why the country was considering building an atomic power plant there. David Ben-Gurion said that if you did not have atomic energy, you were not a modern nation. That was the mind-set the United States had created and sold all over the world.

The AEC had the dual role of promoting and regulating nuclear power, but promotion was their priority. It suppressed documents from staff that raised safety questions. Safety was not discussed in public during the euphoria of the 1960s, when everyone and their uncle were ordering nuclear power plants. There is no such thing as peaceful atoms. The road to the atomic bomb is the nuclear power plant, which has also led to confrontations with nations such as Iran and North Korea, who are just implementing the program that America sold to the world. It is the height of hypocrisy and arrogance that America expects the world to support its attempts to stop countries from building bombs when it is promoting nuclear power.

There has been one constant throughout: nuclear power has never been economical, and it never will be. Even with the latest improvements, the cost overrun is about one or two billion dollars. Thirty years ago, when we went on a nuclear binge, nuclear power was the alternative source of power. There were no alternative technologies that were sustainable and clean. Affordable wind power and solar power were still to come. The situation now is entirely different.

There is no antinuclear movement today. There are, of course, a few souls who gather every once in a while to say the same old things to each other, but the antinuclear movement has lost all connection with the American people. Three Mile Island set the nuclear industry back for twenty or thirty years, but there are still 150 reactors in the United States that can cause major destruction if there is an earthquake or human accident. Every ten years, there has been an accident of some kind, and there is no reason to think that the cycle has ended.

Too much of what comes from the antinuclear movement has been negative. Instead, to persuade the entire nation, the movement must unite with other environmentalists to agree that nuclear power is as much an existential threat to human-kind as climate change. It also needs to make a positive case. It needs collectively to inform people that there are alternative sources of energy and it is not simply a matter of choosing between carbon and plutonium.

Every scientist can be a spokesperson. The world has to count on people with knowledge not just to write doctoral papers but to speak out and to speak to the layperson—to talk about aspects of nuclear power that the average American can relate to. The average American does not think a power plant that has operated for twenty-five years without accident will suddenly become a killer. What does impress people is telling them in plain English that there is thirty years' worth of spent fuel, or radioactive trash, piled up in their backyards that no one knows where to store safely. The trash sits in a swimming pool, which if it loses water will cause a fire that is the equivalent of a bomb in power and scale. The strongest argument for shutting down nuclear reactors is that it is immoral to produce more radioactive trash if no one knows what to do with it other than to hand the problem down to future generations—to sweep the dirt under the carpet. Moreover, no one has ever talked about the cost of monitoring this trash in the future.

Nonetheless, I am an optimist. Solar and wind energy are now more cost-effective, and many states require that they be implemented. While it is necessary to talk about radioactive trash and that every nuclear power plant raises electricity rates, the antinuclear movement must also spend some of its energy advocating solar energy. Then maybe we can win.

20

The Nuclear Age and Future Generations

Helen Caldicott

In 2007, Arjun Makhijani published a remarkable study called *Carbon-Free and Nuclear-Free: A Roadmap for U.S. Energy Policy*. Originating from a symposium I had organized and a presentation given there by David Freeman, it showed that America could indeed be both carbon- and nuclear-free by 2050 by converting to alternative sources of energy. Solar panels could be installed on all houses as they have been in much of Germany, and, with enough wind west of the Mississippi to supply three times the energy America needs, windmills could be installed across the country. Yet, with a pathetic Congress in Washington and a president captive to corporations in the White House, nothing less than a revolution can realize this vision in the next fifty years.

When I first came to the United States in 1978, almost every American I spoke to said it was better to be dead than red. In other words, they would rather have had a nuclear war than be Communist. Against this backdrop of mass psychosis, Physicians for Social Responsibility and I recruited

23,000 doctors in 153 chapters and trained them to engage with the media, which was soon deluged with information. The media's reaction was to question why doctors should be involved in what was essentially a political issue, not a medical issue. Our response was that it *was* a medical issue because nuclear war would destroy the human race.

We continued to organize symposia across the nation, which garnered further attention. People began to listen. The archbishop of Boston became concerned, having woken up one morning, seen a map in the *Boston Globe* showing what might happen in the event of nuclear attack (everyone vaporized in a five-mile radius; third-degree burns out to twenty miles; three thousand square miles in flames), and said, "I don't think Jesus would like this." Celebrities such as Lily Tomlin and Sally Field joined us, too—a boon as far as the media was concerned, because who wants to watch an Australian doctor in a tweed suit talking about the medical effects of nuclear war?

After five years, 80 percent of Americans were opposed to nuclear war, including Ronald Reagan. I remember coming out from a long meeting with the president, in which I felt I had not persuaded him, only to later hear him say that nuclear war must never be fought and can never be won. He then started working with Mikhail Gorbachev, who himself had seen doctors on television talking about the medical consequences of nuclear war. I remember, too, asking House Speaker Tip O'Neill to play our film *The Last Epidemic* on every monitor in Congress, and he did. He later said that supporting the nuclear weapons freeze was one of the most important moments of his career.

We organized a demonstration in Central Park, which turned out to be one of the largest demonstrations in American history. More than a million attended, including black lesbians from Harlem, Southern Christian Baptists, and Mormons from Salt Lake City. Reagan may have returned to talking about Star Wars and missile defense in America's interests but by then almost the entire population of America supported an end to nuclear weapons. We had created a revolution—a peaceful revolution that contributed to the end of the Cold War.

It was education that did the trick. As Thomas Jefferson said, "An informed democracy will behave in a responsible fashion." But the younger generations who now spend all their time tweeting and texting on their cell phones are not informed; they do not understand what they will inherit from the nuclear age, and that troubles me. Not only is there the possibility of future nuclear accidents, they will inherit massive quantities of radioactive waste, which no one knows where to store. This waste will leak, contaminating food and water, and ultimately induce epidemics of cancer and irreparable damage to our genes. Imagine our descendants waking up to radioactive food, to radioactive breast milk, to babies deformed because they were exposed to radiation in utero, to children diagnosed with cancer at the age of six. Meanwhile, the nuclear industry is only concerned with building further power plants; they are arrogant enough not to show any interest in cleaning up after themselves or in the harm that radioactive waste will cause in the future.

This harm encompasses genetic mutations, almost all of which cause disease and are found in recessive genes (most mutations in dominant genes are lethal). The problem is, as Hermann Joseph Muller's Nobel Prize–winning experiments on drosophila fruit flies have shown, it can take twenty generations for mutations to manifest themselves as diabetes or cystic fibrosis or any of the six thousand diseases now known to be genetically inherited. From a medical perspective, therefore, it is absurd to conclude that because there have been no signs of genetic abnormalities directly caused by the nuclear bombs of Hiroshima and Nagasaki, the survivors have not suffered any damage to their genes.

The Japanese government has proposed allowing doses as high as two rems per year to schoolchildren, claiming the risk is low. An exposure at this level over five years—a total of ten rems—for a girl starting at age five would create a cancer incidence of around 3 percent, according to risk estimates in the *BEIR VII* report. Around three out of every one hundred girls—for boys the risk is lower—would develop cancer, and in one of those three, the cancer could be attributed to radiation exposure. The terrible impact, however, is greater than this. Imagine the fear and the guilt parents would feel knowing that their child might develop cancer as a result of such exposure, especially given the long latency period of most cancers. The Pentagon understood this when it evaluated the extent of contamination produced by the July 1946 underground nuclear bomb test at Bikini Atoll. Their report read:

> Of the survivors in contaminated areas, some would be doomed of radiation sickness in hours, some in days, some in years. But, these areas, irregular in size and shape, as wind and topography might form them, would have no visible boundaries. No survivor could be certain he was not among the doomed and so added to every terror of the moment thousands would be stricken with the fear of death and the uncertainty of its time of arrival.

This is what is happening around Fukushima. This is what happened around Chornobyl.

We are in a serious predicament. We are facing the end of life on this planet. I once asked Carl Sagan if he thought there was any other intelligent life in the universe. He paused and said, "No. Because if any species had reached our stage of evolution, they would have destroyed themselves."

We certainly seem to be bent on self-destruction. America and Russia own 97 percent of the hydrogen bombs in the world. Each country has about one thousand on hair-trigger alert, and about one thousand hackers attempt to infiltrate the Pentagon computers in a single day. The United States spends trillions of dollars on what is in effect socialized killing while the nation does not have a free health care system available like most civilized societies.

Global warming is also upon us. In Australia, we have had the hottest days we have ever had. I live in the middle of a forest of eucalyptus trees that explode with the heat. Ash falls from the sky as bushfires burn, while other parts of the country suffer severe floods. Meanwhile, we continue to export our coal to China, where it is burned, causing so much pollution that people find it difficult to breathe and are buying bottles of oxygen. We continue to manufacture more and more plastic, even when there is an island in the Pacific twice the size of Texas made entirely of plastic trash, which causes both intestinal obstruction and carcinogenic BPA and phthalate poisoning in the fish that feed on it and the birds that feed on the fish. We continue to allow fracking, which irreparably harms the environment. And all the while, the true god is money. All anyone believes in anymore is making more money, which is killing Earth.

Earth is gravely ill, and we must all now be physicians to the ailing planet. Otherwise we leave our children nothing. We can, however, stop global warming. We can stop coal mining. We can stop fracking. We can stop wasting electricity. We can do better than to manufacture plutonium just so that we can boil water at any time of the day. We can cover over parking lots around the nation with solar panels and have solar-powered electric cars. We can turn to solar, wind, and geothermal power for our energy needs.

Our sense of entitlement is extraordinary. We waste up to 30 percent of our electricity, yet ask most people where their electricity comes from and they do not have a clue. Nor would they know that if, for instance, we were all to stop using clothes dryers, it would save almost the same amount of energy as that produced by nuclear power. What we need to do is to educate people through the media; to give doctors and scientists a platform to analyze and expound upon the data; to teach people to think about the way we live and the consequences of nuclear power; and above all, to seriously think about how to save our children. America has become as wealthy as it is not only because of its natural resources but also because of the ingenuity of its people. America can easily show Earth what an energy-responsible nation can do, and it could take pride in its achievements. But for that, there needs to be a revolution, and that revolution has to come from you.

Notes

INTRODUCTION BY HELEN CALDICOTT

1. "Japan Sat on U.S. Radiation Maps Showing Immediate Fallout from Nuke Crisis," *Japan Times*, June 18, 2012.

2. E. Bagge, A. Bjelle, S. Eden, and A. Svanborg, "Osteoarthritis in the Elderly: Clinical and Radiological Findings in 79 and 85 Year Olds," *Annals of the Rheumatic Diseases* 50, no. 8 (1991): 535–39. Epub 1991/08/01.

3. Ibid.

4. A.V. Yablokov, V.B. Nesterenko, A.V. Nesterenko, and J.D. Sherman-Nevinger, *Chernobyl: Consequences of the Catastrophe for People and the Environment* (New York: Wiley, 2010).

5. Fukushima Health Management, *Proceedings of the 15th Prefectural Oversight Committee Meeting for Fukushima Health Management Survey*, Fukushima, Japan, 2014.

6. A.P. Møller and T.A. Mousseau, "The Effects of Low-Dose Radiation: Soviet Science, the Nuclear Industry—and Independence?," *Significance* 10, no. 1 (2013): 14–19.

5: THE CONTAMINATION OF JAPAN WITH RADIOACTIVE CESIUM BY STEVEN STARR

1. For example, the Norwegian Institute for Air Research estimates that the destroyed nuclear reactors at Fukushima released

2.5 times more radioactive xenon-133 gas than the destruction of the nuclear reactor at Chornobyl. Xenon-133 has a half-life of about five days, so in two months most of it had disappeared from the environment. But the winds from Fukushima carried a giant cloud of xenon-133 directly over the Tokyo metropolitan area, where (according to the Japan Chemical Analysis Center) it averaged 1,300 atomic disintegrations per second in every cubic meter of air from March 14 through March 22, 2011. The Japanese government chose not to warn people in Tokyo to take any precautions.

2. This is not to diminish the importance of other long-lived radionuclides released by catastrophic nuclear accidents, such as strontium-90 and plutonium, which can affect living things in equally bad or even worse ways. But there appears to be proportionally much less of these radionuclides released than cesium-137 in reactor accidents, so the emphasis in this chapter is on radioactive cesium.

3. Cesium becomes a gas at 1,240 degrees Fahrenheit (at one atmosphere of pressure), whereas fuel rods heat to the point of rupture at about 1,500 degrees Fahrenheit and ignite at 3,300 degrees Fahrenheit. The buildup of gas pressure inside the rod causes it to rupture (the zirconium cladding bursts). The zirconium cladding on spent fuel rods will react exothermically when exposed to air and heated to around 1,800 degrees Fahrenheit, creating a catastrophic fire with consequences potentially worse than a reactor meltdown. (B. Alvarez, "What About the Spent Fuel?," *Bulletin of the Atomic Scientists*, January–February 2002, 45–47.)

4. This fallout is most concentrated by rainfall that washes it from the sky, which tends to concentrate it in an irregular fashion, accounting for its patchy deposition.

5. The distribution of cesium-137 tends to be uneven, of course, but it is found in everything from the trees, which produce radioactive smoke when their firewood is used for cooking

and heating, to all varieties of plant and animal tissues. Daily exposure to small amounts of radionuclides in such environments (mostly cesium-137) is virtually unavoidable because they enter the body via up to 94 percent of foodstuffs (V. Nesterenko and A. Nesterenko, "Decorporation of Chernobyl Radionuclides," in *Chernobyl: Consequences of the Catastrophe for People and the Environment*, in *Annals of the New York Academy of Sciences*, vol. 1181 (Boston: Blackwell Publishing on behalf of the New York Academy of Sciences, 2009), viii, 304.

6. Plants and animals in both aquatic and terrestrial ecosystems tend to accumulate cesium as they would potassium. This is especially true for terrestrial organisms rich in potassium, such as fungi and berries. Cesium uptake in plants can be somewhat limited by the addition of potassium fertilizers; it is also taken up less in aquatic systems where waters are murkier.

7. A. Madrigal, "Chernobyl Exclusion Zone Radioactive Longer Than Expected," Wired.com, December 15, 2009.

8. I realize that these are considered "old" terms to describe radioactivity, but they are the most straightforward and easiest to understand for most people. I think that the numerous changes in terminology in radiological science have in part been done to obscure such meanings from nontechnical audiences.

9. There are highly radioactive naturally occurring radionuclides, such as radon and its daughter product, polonium, which have very short half-lives. These are not commonly found in foodstuffs because they self-destruct long before they can make it into the food chains.

10. The 88 curies per gram includes the decay process of cesium-137 to barium-137m, in which the barium-137m emits high-powered gamma radiation. Barium-137m has a half-life of not quite three minutes.

11. The models use weighting factors to multiply the estimated biological effects of various atomic particles (twenty times for alpha particles) and the given tissue where it resides. But the

multiplication is quickly negated by many orders of magnitude when the dose given to a tiny cluster of cells is averaged over the organ system or body area in which the tiny cluster of cells resides.

12. R. Alvarez, J. Beyea, K. Janberg, J. Kang, E. Lyman, A. Macfarlane, G. Thompson, and F. von Hippel, "Reducing the Hazards from Stored Spent Power-Reactor Fuel in the United States," *Science and Global Security* 11 (2003): 7.

13. "The Big Picture," RT.com, May 17, 2011, retrieved from http://www.youtube.com/watch?v=xEFtfkJc4kM.

14. These scientists declined my request to republish the image here, but it can be found online as slide number 25 in Gayle Sugiyama and John Nasstrom, "Overview of the NARAC Modeling During the Response to the Fukushima Dai-ichi Power Plant Emergency," International Workshop on Source Term Estimation Methods for Estimating the Atmospheric Radiation Release from the Fukushima Daiichi Nuclear Power Plant, February 22–24, 2012, http://www.ral.ucar.edu/nsap/events/fukushima/documents/Session1_Briefing3-Sugiyama.pdf.

15. One millisievert per year is similar to current U.S. radiation safety exposure standards.

16. This figure was provided to me by the former Japanese ambassador to Switzerland Mitsuhei Murata, who obtained these figures from government officials in Fukushima Prefecture.

17. M. Fackler, "Japan's Nuclear Refugees, Still Stuck in Limbo," *New York Times*, October 1, 2013.

18. Comments by the Committee to Bridge the Gap, NIRS, PSR Los Angeles, and the Southern California Federation of Scientists on the National Council on Radiation Protection and Measurements's draft report SC 5-1, "Approach to Optimizing Decision Making for Late-Phase Recovery from Nuclear or Radiological Terrorism Incidents," April 2013.

19. A. Makhijani, "The Use of Reference Man in Radiation Protection Standards with Recommendations for Guidance and

Change," Institute for Energy and Environmental Research, December 2008.

20. Ibid.

21. These conversions are made through the multiplication of hypothesized "radiation weighting factors" times the absorbed dose in order to obtain the equivalent dose, and through the subsequent multiplication of hypothesized "tissue weighting factors" times the equivalent dose to obtain a total effective dose. "Effective dose coefficients" are also calculated and then used to calculate an internal dose that becomes a "committed" dose, averaged over time, after the radionuclide enters the body.

22. Committee Examining Radiation Risks of Internal Emitters, London, "Report of the Committee Examining Radiation Risks of Internal Emitters (CERRIE)," October 2004.

23. Significant quantities of cesium-137 may also be making their way into human bodies through the inhalation of radioactive smoke. This is because in most rural homes of Belarus and Ukraine, cooking and heating is done with wood, and the wood in contaminated areas has become radioactive. Burning the wood releases its radioactivity. Vassili Nesterenko, a prominent Soviet physicist who lived in Belarus (he died in 2008), stated that chimneys in these households became "miniature nuclear reactors" after constantly burning radioactive wood.

24. ICRP, "Application of the Commission's Recommendations to the Protection of People Living in Long-Term Contaminated Areas After a Nuclear Accident or a Radiation Emergency," *Annals of the ICRP* 39, no. 3 (2009).

25. Y. Bandazhevsky, "Chronic Cs-137 Incorporation in Children's Organs," *Swiss Medical Weekly* 133, no. 35–36 (2003): 488–90.

26. There is an excellent documentary, *Nuclear Controversies* by Wladimir Tchertkoff, that tells much of this story and includes an interview with Dr. Bandazhevsky while he was under house arrest.

27. The Institute of Radiation Safety "BELRAD" website, "General Overview" (www.belrad-institute.org/UK/doku.php).

28. A. Yablokov, V. Nesterenko, and A. Nesterenko, "Chernobyl: Consequences of the Catastrophe for People and the Environment," in *Annals of the New York Academy of Sciences* vol. 1181 (Boston: Blackwell Publishing on behalf of the New York Academy of Sciences, 2009), viii, 42.

29. United Nations Development Program, *Belarus: Choices for the Future* (Minsk: National Human Development Report, 2000), 32, http://hdr.undp.org/sites/default/files/belarus_2000_en.pdf.

30. J. Vidal, "UN Accused of Ignoring 500,000 Chernobyl Deaths," *The Guardian*, March 24, 2006.

31. Ibid.

32. International Physicians for the Prevention of Nuclear War, "Health Effects of Chernobyl: 25 Years After the Reactor Catastrophe," April 2011.

33. Ibid.

34. Nuclear power plants produce electricity using the same principle as coal- and gas-fired power plants. They produce large amounts of heat in order to boil water and produce steam, which then is used to power the turbines that generate electricity. Nuclear power plants were not invented to make electricity. They were designed to produce plutonium to be used in nuclear weapons. Every thousand-megawatt commercial nuclear plant that uses uranium for fuel produces enough plutonium every year to build about forty nuclear weapons.

10: WHAT THE WORLD HEALTH ORGANIZATION, INTERNATIONAL ATOMIC ENERGY AGENCY, AND INTERNATIONAL COMMISSION ON RADIOLOGICAL PROTECTION HAVE FALSIFIED BY ALEXEY V. YABLOKOV

References

Arynchyn, A.N., and L.A. Ospennikova. "Lens Opacities in Children of Belarus Affected by the Chernobyl Accident." In *Recent Research Activities on the Chernobyl Accident in*

Belarus, Ukraine, and Russia, ed. T. Imanaka, 168–77. Kyoto: Kyoto University, 1998.

Bennet, Burton, Michael Repacholi, and Zhanat Carr, eds. *Health Effects of the Chernobyl Accident and Special Health Care Programmes: Report of the Chernobyl Forum Expert Group "Health".* Geneva: World Health Organization, 2006.

Broda, R. "Gamma Spectroscopy Analysis of Hot Particles from the Chernobyl Fallout." *Acta Physica Polonica* B18, no. 10 (1987): 935–50.

Fairlie, I., and D. Sumner. *The Other Report on Chernobyl (TORCH).* Berlin: Altner Combecher Foundation, 2006.

Grodzinsky, D.M. "Ecological and Biological Consequences of the Chernobyl Accident." In *Chernobyl Catastrophe: History, Social, Economics, Geochemical, Medical and Biological Consequences,* ed. V.G. Bar'yakhtar, 290–315. Kiev: Naukova Dumka, 1995.

Koerblein, A. "Studies of Pregnancy Outcome Following the Chernobyl Accident." In *ECRR: Chernobyl 20 Years On: Health Effects of the Chernobyl Accident,* ed. C.C. Busby and A.V. Yablokov, 227–43. Aberystwyth: Green Audit Books, 2006.

Koerblein, A. "Einfluss der Form der Dosis-Wirkungsbeziehung auf das Leukämierisiko." *Strahlentelex,* nos. 524–25 (2008): 8–10.

Kryvolutsky, D.A. *Change in Ecology and Biodiversity After a Nuclear Disaster in the Southern Urals.* Sofia: Pensoft, 1998.

Lyaginskaya, A.M., A.R. Tukov, V.A. Osypov, and O.N. Prokhorova. "Genetic Effects on Chernobyl's Liquidators." *Radiation Biology Radioecology* 47, no. 2 (2007): 188–95.

Malko, M.V. "Assessment of the Medical Consequences of the Chernobyl Accident." In *The Health Effects on the Human Victims of the Chernobyl Catastrophe,* ed. I.P. Blokov, 194–235. Amsterdam: Greenpeace International, 2007.

Petoussi-Henss, N., et al. "Conversion Coefficients for

Radiological Protection Quantities for External Radiation Exposures." *Annals of the ICRP* 40, no. 2–5 (2010).

Scherb, H., and K. Voigt. "The Human Sex Odds at Birth After the Atmospheric Atomic Bomb Tests, After Chernobyl, and in the Vicinity of Nuclear Facilities." *Environmental Science and Pollution Research* 18, no. 5 (June 2011): 697–707.

Sinkko, K., H. Aaltonen, R. Mustonen, T.K. Taipale, and J. Juutilainen. *Airborne Radioactivity in Finland after the Chernobyl Accident in 1986*, Report STUK-A56. Helsinki: Finnish Center for Radiation and Nuclear Safety, 1987.

Sperling, K., H. Neitzel, and H. Scherb. "Evidence for an Increase in Trisomy 21 (Down Syndrome) in Europe After the Chernobyl Reactor Accident." *Genetic Epidemiology* 36, no. 1 (2012): 48–55.

Tscheglov, A.I. *Biogeochemistry of Technogenic Radionuclides in the Forest Ecosystems*. Moscow: Nauka, 1999.

Yablokov, A.V., V.B. Nesterenko, and A.V. Nesterenko. "Chernobyl: Consequences of the Catastrophe for People and the Environment." *Annals of the New York Academy of Sciences* 1181 (2009).

11: CONGENITAL MALFORMATIONS IN RIVNE, UKRAINE BY WLADIMIR WERTELECKI

1. A unit of absorbed radiation equivalent to one joule of energy per kilogram of matter.

References

Dancause, Kelsey Needham, Lyubov Yevtushok, Serhiy Lapchenko, Ihor Shumlyansky, Genadiy Shevchenko, Wladimir Wertelecki, and Ralph M. Garruto. "Chronic Radiation Exposure in the Rivne-Polissia Region of Ukraine: Implications for Birth Defects." *American Journal of Human Biology* 22, no. 5 (2010): 667–74, doi:10.1002/ajhb.21063.

Wertelecki, Wladimir, Lyubov Yevtushok, Natalia Zymak-
    Zakutnia, Bin Wang, Zoriana Sosyniuk, Serhiy Lapchenko,
    and Holly H. Hobart. "Blastopathies and Microcephaly
    in a Chornobyl Impacted Region of Ukraine." *Congenital
    Anomalies*, January 13, 2014, doi:10.1111/cga.12051 (online
    publication ahead of print publication).

18: CANCER RISK FROM EXPOSURE TO LOW LEVELS OF IONIZING RADIATION BY HERBERT ABRAMS

References

Beyea, J., and M. Bricker. "Risks of Exposure to Low-Level
    Radiation." *Bulletin of the Atomic Scientists* 68 (2012).

About the Contributors

HERBERT ABRAMS is emeritus professor of radiology at Stanford University and a member of the Biological Effects of Ionizing Radiation (BEIR) Committee of the National Academy of Sciences.

ROBERT ALVAREZ is a senior scholar at the Institute for Policy Studies.

DAVID BRENNER is the Higgins Professor of Radiation Biophysics at the College of Physicians and Surgeons at Columbia University.

IAN FAIRLIE is a radiation biologist and an independent consultant on radiation risks. He is also the former scientific secretary to the British government's Committee Examining Radiation Risks of Internal Emitters.

CINDY FOLKERS is a specialist in radiation and health for Beyond Nuclear.

DAVID FREEMAN is the former chairman of the Tennessee Valley Authority and the former general manager of the Los Angeles Department of Water and Power, the New York Power Authority, and the Sacramento Municipal Utility District.

ARNOLD GUNDERSEN is a nuclear engineer at Fairewinds Energy Education.

KEVIN KAMPS is a specialist in high-level waste management and transportation at Beyond Nuclear.

NAOTO KAN is the former prime minister of Japan.

HIROAKI KOIDE is a specialist in radiation safety and control at the Kyoto University Research Reactor Institute.

DAVID LOCHBAUM is the director of the Union of Concerned Scientists Nuclear Safety Project.

AKIO MATSUMURA is the founder of the Global Forum of Spiritual and Parliamentary Leaders.

TIMOTHY MOUSSEAU is a professor of biological sciences at the University of South Carolina.

MARY OLSON is the director of the Southeast Office of the Nuclear Information and Resource Service.

HISAKO SAKIYAMA is a former senior researcher at the National Institute of Radiological Sciences. She was also a member of the Fukushima Nuclear Accident Independent Investigation Commission.

STEVEN STARR is a senior scientist at Physicians for Social Responsibility and the director of the Clinical Laboratory Science Program at the University of Missouri.

WLADIMIR WERTELECKI is the president of the board of the OMNI-Net Ukraine child development programs and an adjunct professor of biomedical anthropology at the State University of New York.

STEVEN WING is an associate professor of epidemiology at the Gillings School of Global Public Health at the University of North Carolina.

ALEXEY V. YABLOKOV is a member of the Russian Academy of Sciences.

About the Editor

The world's leading spokesperson for the antinuclear movement, DR. HELEN CALDICOTT is the co-founder of Physicians for Social Responsibility, a nominee for the Nobel Peace Prize, and the 2003 winner of the Lannan Prize for Cultural Freedom. Both the Smithsonian Institute and *Ladies' Home Journal* have named her one of the Most Influential Women of the Twentieth Century. In 2001, she founded the Nuclear Policy Research Institute, which later became Beyond Nuclear, in Washington, D.C. The author of *The New Nuclear Danger*, *War in Heaven* (with Craig Eisendrath), *Nuclear Power Is Not the Answer*, and *Loving This Planet* (all published by The New Press), she is currently president of the Helen Caldicott Foundation/NuclearFreePlanet.org.

Publishing in the Public Interest

Thank you for reading this book published by The New Press. The New Press is a nonprofit, public interest publisher. New Press books and authors play a crucial role in sparking conversations about the key political and social issues of our day.

We hope you enjoyed this book and that you will stay in touch with The New Press. Here are a few ways to stay up to date with our books, events, and the issues we cover:

- Sign up at www.thenewpress.com/subscribe to receive updates on New Press authors and issues and to be notified about local events
- Like us on Facebook: www.facebook.com/ newpressbooks
- Follow us on Twitter: www.twitter.com/thenewpress

Please consider buying New Press books for yourself; for friends and family; or to donate to schools, libraries, community centers, prison libraries, and other organizations involved with the issues our authors write about.

The New Press is a 501(c)(3) nonprofit organization. You can also support our work with a tax-deductible gift by visiting www.thenewpress.com/donate.